Severe Community-Acquired Pneumonia

Severe community-acquired pneumonia (sCAP) remains a significant threat to global health, causing immense morbidity and mortality. This book explores recent advances in pathogens, host immunity, and antimicrobial resistance. It presents details on innovative diagnostic techniques, including novel imaging modalities and biomarkers for rapid and accurate diagnosis, and provides up-to-date guidance on therapeutic strategies such as FAST HUGS BID, along with palliative care and rehabilitation, supported by case studies. This practical guide is a ready reckoner for internal medicine residents, pulmonologists, and critical care specialists.

Key Features:

- Presents details on preventative measures, including vaccination strategies and public health interventions.
- Provides a comprehensive and up-to-date current resource companion for Internal Medicine Residency, Pulmonology and Critical Care Consultants.
- Offers a roadmap to navigate the ever-changing landscape of severe community-acquired pneumonia, including newer diagnostic methods, immunology, and up-to-date management.

Severe Community-Acquired Pneumonia

Gurmeet Singh

CRC Press
Taylor & Francis Group
Boca Raton London New York

CRC Press is an imprint of the
Taylor & Francis Group, an **informa** business

Designed cover image: Shutterstock id: 2395659735

First edition published 2026
by CRC Press
2385 NW Executive Center Drive, Suite 320, Boca Raton FL 33431

and by CRC Press
4 Park Square, Milton Park, Abingdon, Oxon, OX14 4RN

CRC Press is an imprint of Taylor & Francis Group, LLC

© 2026 Gurmeet Singh

ISBN: 978-1-041-04708-7 (hbk)
ISBN: 978-1-041-04707-0 (pbk)
ISBN: 978-1-003-62950-4 (ebk)

DOI: 10.1201/9781003629504

Typeset in Caslon
by SPi Technologies India Pvt Ltd (Straive)

Access the Support Material: https://www.routledge.com/9781003629504

This Book is Dedicated to My Family.

They had a decisive influence on the course of my life. To the memory of my late grandfather, Harchand Singh, my late grandmother, Jaswant Kaur, my late mother, Kuljit Kaur. To my father, Manmohan Singh, my wife, Simarjeet Kaur, my daughters, Milandeep Kaur and Harshavin Kaur, and my son, Shanndeep Singh. To my sister, Hardeep Kaur and my brothers, Bhupinder Singh and Jadbinder Singh.

Contents

Preface

Severe community-acquired pneumonia (sCAP) remains a major challenge in clinical medicine, demanding timely diagnosis, appropriate antimicrobial therapy, and multidisciplinary care. The evolving microbial landscape, rising antimicrobial resistance, and complexity of critically ill patients highlight the need for continuous learning and updated clinical guidance.

This monograph, *Severe Community-Acquired Pneumonia*, consists of 12 chapters that provide comprehensive, evidence-based updates on sCAP. It covers key clinical aspects from etiology and pathogenesis to diagnosis, treatment, and prognosis. The final chapter presents a series of challenging real-world cases, offering practical insights to complement the core content.

I extend my sincere gratitude to doctors and nurses at Cipto Mangunkusumo General Hospital (RSCM), Universitas Indonesia, especially staff from the Respirology and Critical Care Division Internal Medicine Department, ICU/HCU, and interventional pulmonology teams.

I would like to thank the leadership and colleagues at Cipto Mangunkusumo Hospital and MRCCC Siloam Hospital, as well as the Dean of the Faculty of Medicine, Universitas Indonesia, for their support in bringing this book to completion. I would also like to express my sincere appreciation to Robiatul Adawiyah, MD, PhD (Department of Parasitology, Faculty of Medicine, Universitas Indonesia), Muhamad Yanuar, MD (Department of Radiology, Universitas Indonesia), and Hariadi Hadibrata, MD (Siloam Hospital) for their generous contribution of clinical figures that significantly enhanced the clarity and educational value of this monograph.

I'm especially grateful to my research assistants, Steffi Cong Andi Nata and Nova Bornida Fauzi, for their invaluable help in developing the content and sourcing reference materials. My deepest appreciation also goes to the patients and families who permitted the inclusion of their cases in this book.

It is my hope that this work will serve as a useful resource for clinicians, educators, and trainees involved in the care of patients with severe community-acquired pneumonia.

Associate Professor Gurmeet Singh, MD, DM, PhD
Jakarta, Indonesia
May, 2025

Acknowledgment

The development of this monograph would not have been possible without the invaluable support, mentorship, and inspiration from a number of individuals to whom I extend my deepest gratitude.

Faculty Leadership

- Prof. Ari Fahrial Syam, MD, PhD, SpPD-KGEH, MMB, Dean, Faculty of Medicine, Universitas Indonesia
- Prof. Ratna Sitompul, MD, PhD, SpM(K) Former Dean, Faculty of Medicine, Universitas Indonesia

Senior Professors and Mentors

From the Department of Internal Medicine, Cipto Mangunkusumo Hospital, Universitas Indonesia:

- Prof. Czeresna Heriawan Soejono, MD, PhD, SpPD-KGer, M.Epid, MPH
- Prof. H. Dadang Makmun, MD, PhD, SpPD-KGEH
- Prof. Imam Subekti, MD, PhD, SpPD-KEMD

Division of Respirology and Critical Illness, Department of Internal Medicine, Cipto Mangunkusumo Hospital, Universitas Indonesia:

- Prof. Zulkifli Amin, MD, PhD, SpPD-KPMK, FICCP
- Prof. Cleopas Martin Rumende, MD, PhD, SpPD-KPMK, FICCP

- Dr. Ceva W. Pitoyo, MD, SpPD-KPMK, KIC
- Dr. Anna Uyainah Z.N., MD, SpPD-KPMK, MARS *(In memoriam)*

Their lifelong dedication to internal medicine and clinical education continues to inspire this generation and many more to come.

International Inspiration

I would also like to express my deepest appreciation to:

- Prof. Surendra K. Sharma, MD, PhD, JC Bose Fellow, ATSF Professor of Medicine, Department of Medicine, All India Institute of Medical Sciences (AIIMS), New Delhi, India Fellow of the American Thoracic Society (ATSF) JC Bose National Fellow, Government of India for his exemplary leadership in pulmonary and critical care medicine. His academic contributions and lifelong commitment to advancing global respiratory medicine continue to be a source of inspiration for physicians and researchers worldwide.

About the Author

Gurmeet Singh is a leading authority in the field of pneumonia, particularly severe community-acquired pneumonia, with more than 15 years of experience in respirology and critical care medicine. His expertise also includes chronic obstructive pulmonary disease (COPD), acute respiratory distress syndrome (ARDS), and lung cancer, as well as advanced interventional procedures such as bronchoscopy and medical thoracoscopy. He practices at both RSUPN Dr. Cipto Mangunkusumo, Indonesia's National Hospital, and MRCCC Siloam Semanggi (Mochtar Riady Comprehensive Cancer Center), one of Indonesia's premier cancer hospitals. Dr. Singh serves as the Head of the Respirology and Critical Illness Division at Universitas Indonesia and leads the Jakarta Branch of the Indonesian Respiratory Society. In addition to his clinical roles, he is a lecturer in the Department of Internal Medicine at Universitas Indonesia and he was recently (June 2025) promoted to Associate Professor 2025. He has authored numerous scientific publications and is a regular speaker at national and international forums. His previous book, *Challenging Cases in Respirology and Critical Care* (Springer Nature, 2025), showcases his case-based clinical approach. This book, *Severe Community-Acquired Pneumonia*, provides comprehensive, evidence-based guidance for clinicians managing this life-threatening respiratory condition.

CHAPTER 1

Introduction to Severe Community-Acquired Pneumonia

1.1 Introduction

Severe community-acquired pneumonia (sCAP) is a critical and often life-threatening condition that poses a significant challenge to healthcare systems worldwide. According to the Infectious Diseases Society of America (IDSA) and the American Thoracic Society (ATS), sCAP requires prompt recognition and intervention to mitigate its high morbidity and mortality. As one of the leading infectious causes of morbidity and mortality, sCAP demands accurate diagnosis, effective management, and timely intervention to improve outcomes and reduce the burden on healthcare resources.[1]

1.2 Pneumonia Scoring

Pneumonia scoring systems are essential tools for assessing the severity of community-acquired pneumonia (CAP) and guiding clinical decision-making. These

 DOI:10.1201/9781003629504-1

scoring systems help clinicians identify patients at higher risk for adverse outcomes, determine the need for hospitalization, and select appropriate therapeutic strategies.[2,3]

1.2.1 CURB-65

The CURB-65 score evaluates five clinical criteria:

1. Confusion.
2. Urea ≥7 mmol/L or ≥20 mg/dl.
3. Respiratory rate ≥30 breaths/minute.
4. Blood pressure (systolic <90 mmHg or diastolic ≤60 mmHg).
5. Age ≥65 years.

Each criterion scores one point, and the total score stratifies patients into low, moderate, or high-risk categories for mortality and guides decisions regarding outpatient versus inpatient care.[2]

1.2.2 PSI (Pneumonia Severity Index)

The Pneumonia Severity Index (PSI) is a more comprehensive scoring system that includes factors such as age, comorbidities, physical examination findings, laboratory results, and radiographic data. It categorizes patients into five risk classes, with higher classes indicating greater risk of mortality and a stronger recommendation for inpatient or intensive care management.[3]

1.2.3 ATS/IDSA 2019 Criteria

The 2019 ATS/IDSA guidelines provide specific major and minor criteria for defining sCAP and determining the need for intensive care unit (ICU) admission. The presence of either one major criterion or three or more minor criteria suggests the need for ICU-level care.[1]

1.2.3.1 Major Criteria

1. Septic shock requiring vasopressors.
2. Respiratory failure requiring mechanical ventilation.

1.2.3.2 Minor Criteria

1. Respiratory rate ≥30 breaths/minute.
2. PaO2/FiO2 ratio ≤250.
3. Multilobar infiltrates.
4. Confusion or altered mental status.
5. Uremia (BUN ≥20 mg/dL).
6. Leukopenia (WBC <4,000 cells/μL).
7. Thrombocytopenia (platelets <100,000/μL).
8. Hypothermia (core temperature <36°C).
9. Hypotension requiring aggressive fluid resuscitation.

These scoring systems and guidelines are invaluable for optimizing resource utilization and improving patient outcomes by tailoring management strategies to disease severity.[1-3]

1.3 Epidemiology

Severe community-acquired pneumonia accounts for a substantial proportion of hospital admissions and is associated with high mortality rates, particularly among older adults, immunocompromised individuals, and those with underlying comorbidities. The estimated worldwide incidence of community-acquired pneumonia varies between 1.5 and 14 cases per 1000 person-years and is affected by geography, season, and population characteristics.[4] In the US, the annual incidence is 248 cases per 100,000 adults, with higher rates observed in older age groups. Pneumonia is the eighth-leading cause of death overall, and the leading cause of death from infectious diseases. The mortality rate reaches up to 23% among patients admitted to the ICU for severe pneumonia.[5] Two large, monocentre and multicentre observational studies from Spain and the United States of America (USA) recently confirmed such an increased mortality. Overall mortality due to sCAP was 20% higher when patients presented with either shock (22% higher) or invasive mechanical ventilation (25% higher), or both

(30% higher). Furthermore, sCAP is one of the most common causes of acute respiratory distress syndrome, and it is reported in ~3% of patients hospitalized with pneumococcal CAP.[6]

Based on the study conducted by Singh et al. in Indonesia, out of a total of n=40 sCAP patients who failed extubation, 75% of the subjects died within the 28-day observation period.[7]

The global burden of sCAP varies geographically due to differences in pathogen prevalence, healthcare infrastructure, and vaccination rates. Advances in global vaccination programs, particularly against *Streptococcus pneumoniae*, have influenced the epidemiology of sCAP, although disparities remain in regions with limited access to vaccines. The annual incidence of CAP ranges from 1.5 to 14 cases per 1,000 individuals, with sCAP comprising 10–20% of hospitalized cases. The in-hospital mortality rate for sCAP is approximately 20–50%, emphasizing the need for timely and effective intervention. Common causative agents include *Streptococcus pneumoniae*, *Legionella pneumophila*, and *Staphylococcus aureus*, though viral pathogens like influenza and SARS-CoV-2 have also emerged as significant contributors.[5]

1.4 Etiology of Community-Acquired Pneumonia

Community-acquired pneumonia is caused by a diverse array of pathogens, including bacteria, viruses, and fungi. The etiology of CAP can vary based on geographic region, season, patient demographics, and underlying health conditions.[8–10]

1.4.1 Bacterial Pathogens

- *Streptococcus pneumoniae*: The most common cause of CAP worldwide, particularly in older adults and those with chronic illnesses.
- *Haemophilus influenzae*: Commonly associated with CAP in patients with chronic obstructive pulmonary disease (COPD).

- *Legionella pneumophila*: Causes Legionnaires' disease, a severe form of CAP often associated with contaminated water sources.
- *Staphylococcus aureus*: Includes methicillin-sensitive and methicillin-resistant strains (MSSA and MRSA), often implicated in post-influenza pneumonia.
- *Klebsiella pneumoniae*: Associated with alcohol use disorder and aspiration risk.[10,11]

1.4.2 Viral Pathogens

- Influenza viruses: A leading cause of viral CAP, particularly during seasonal outbreaks.
- SARS-CoV-2: The causative agent of COVID-19, which has significantly altered the landscape of CAP etiology in recent years.
- Respiratory syncytial virus (RSV): A notable pathogen in older adults and immunocompromised individuals.[12]

1.4.3 Fungal Pathogens

- *Histoplasma capsulatum, Coccidioides immitis*, and *Blastomyces dermatitidis*: Common causes of CAP in endemic regions.
- Opportunistic fungi, such as *Aspergillus* and *Pneumocystis jirovecii*, are more prevalent in immunocompromised patients.[13]

1.4.4 Polymicrobial Infections

- Mixed infections involving bacterial and viral or fungal pathogens are increasingly recognized, particularly in critically ill patients.[14]

1.5 Pathogenesis

The development of sCAP involves a complex interplay between host defense mechanisms and microbial pathogens. The progression to severe disease occurs when the host immune response fails to effectively contain the infection, resulting in widespread inflammation, tissue damage, and mortality.

1.5.1 Pathogen Entry and Initial Host Defense

Microorganisms gain access to the lower respiratory tract through multiple routes, with aspiration from the oropharynx being the most common. Other mechanisms include inhalation of contaminated droplets, hematogenous spread (e.g., from tricuspid endocarditis), or contiguous extension from adjacent infected structures. Once in the lower airways, pathogens encounter the host's primary defense mechanisms, which include mechanical barriers such as nasal hairs, mucociliary clearance, and anatomical structures that prevent pathogen entry into the alveoli. If these defenses fail, alveolar macrophages serve as the first line of immune defense, attempting to eliminate the invading microorganisms.[7]

1.5.2 Inflammatory Response and Disease Progression

When the body initial immune response is insufficient, the infection progresses, leading to an exaggerated immune reaction. The lung's defense mechanisms involve structural, mechanical, secretory, humoral, and cellular components. When these fail to control the infection, alveolar opsonins, surfactants, immunoglobulins (IgG), and the complement system become activated. Neutrophils, monocytes, and macrophages express surface receptors such as sTREM-1, which amplifies inflammatory signaling. This leads to the release of pro-inflammatory cytokines, including interleukin-6 (IL-6), tumor necrosis factor-alpha (TNF-α), and interleukin-1 beta (IL-1β), which mediate systemic and pulmonary inflammation.[7]

The inflammatory cascade triggered by pathogen invasion results in alveolar fluid accumulation, impaired gas exchange, and progressive hypoxemia. In severe cases, the excessive release of pro-inflammatory cytokines contributes to systemic complications such as fever, septic shock, and multi-organ dysfunction. Persistent infection and sustained inflammation further exacerbate lung injury, promoting epithelial dysfunction and vascular endothelial activation.[7]

1.5.3 T-Cell Dysregulation and Lung Injury

T-cell-mediated immunity plays a crucial role in disease progression. The balance between T-cell proliferation and apoptosis is essential for an effective immune response. Excessive apoptosis, triggered by Fas ligand activation and caspase pathways, leads to a reduction in CD4+ T-cell levels, impairing immune regulation. Severe hypoxemia and epithelial dysfunction can induce a strong immune response, further damaging the lung tissue. In cases of acute or chronic lung injury, failure of alveolar epithelial regeneration accelerates disease progression. Regulatory T cells (FoxP3+ T-reg cells) play a critical role in promoting epithelial repair and maintaining immune homeostasis, preventing excessive immunological damage.[7,15]

In sCAP, the failure of immune regulation leads to uncontrolled inflammation, alveolar damage, and systemic complications. The excessive immune response, rather than the direct effect of pathogens alone, significantly contributes to disease severity. Understanding the underlying mechanisms of sCAP pathogenesis is essential for developing targeted therapeutic strategies to mitigate lung injury and improve patient outcomes.[7,15]

1.6 Signs and Symptoms

Patients with sCAP typically present with high fever, chills, and productive cough with purulent sputum; severe dyspnea and hypoxemia often requiring supplemental oxygen or mechanical ventilation; and signs of sepsis, including tachycardia, hypotension, and altered mental status. The presentation can vary widely based on the causative pathogen and host factors, making early and accurate diagnosis essential. Atypical presentations, especially in elderly or immunocompromised patients, may include subtle symptoms such as confusion or functional decline.[12,16]

1.7 Diagnostic Approaches

A systematic approach to diagnosing pneumonia includes clinical evaluation, radiological imaging, and microbiological investigations.[6]

1.7.1 Clinical Presentation

Key symptoms include:

- Cough, often productive with sputum (bacterial pneumonia) or dry (viral or atypical pathogens).
- Fever, chills, and pleuritic chest pain.
- Dyspnea and hypoxia in severe cases.

Physical findings like crackles, bronchial breath sounds, and dullness on percussion can guide suspicion of pneumonia.

1.7.2 Imaging

- Chest X-ray: First-line imaging modality to confirm consolidation or infiltrates. Lobar consolidation suggests bacterial pneumonia, while interstitial patterns are more common in viral infections.
- CT Scan: Offers better resolution for detecting abscesses, cavitations, or atypical patterns in immunocompromised patients.

1.7.3 Microbiological Tests

- Blood cultures: essential in severe pneumonia to detect bacteremia.
- Sputum examination: microscopy, Gram stain, and culture to identify bacterial pathogens.

- Tracheal aspiration: tracheal aspiration is recommended for patients with sCAP who are intubated or mechanically ventilated to identify the causative pathogen.
- Bronchoalveolar lavage (BAL): used in critically ill patients to sample lower respiratory secretions.
- Empiric antimicrobial therapy: should not be withheld while awaiting microbiological results, but results should guide de-escalation or modification of antibiotics when available.

1.7.4 Biomarkers

- Procalcitonin (PCT): helps differentiate bacterial from viral infections.
- C-reactive protein (CRP): reflects inflammation but is less specific.
- sTREM-1 (Soluble Triggering Receptor Expressed on Myeloid Cells-1): is released into the blood and body fluids, making it a biomarker for infection and inflammation severity. Elevated sTREM-1 levels can be detected in plasma, bronchoalveolar lavage (BAL) fluid, and cerebrospinal fluid during infection.

1.8 Rapid Diagnostic Tests

- Urinary Antigen Tests: identify *Legionella pneumophila* and *Streptococcus pneumoniae*.
- Point-of-Care Testing: includes rapid influenza tests and SARS-CoV-2 antigen detection.
- Multiplex Polymerase Chain Reaction (PCR): a rapid and highly sensitive molecular technique for detecting bacterial and viral pathogens. This PCR is particularly useful for identifying *Mycoplasma*

pneumoniae, Chlamydia pneumoniae, Legionella pneumophila, and respiratory viruses such as influenza, SARS-CoV-2, and RSV.

1.9 Special Considerations in Immunocompromised Hosts

- Comprehensive testing for atypical pathogens, including fungal and parasitic agents.
- Biopsies and advanced molecular techniques like next-generation sequencing in non-resolving pneumonia.

Early recognition of sCAP is crucial for initiating appropriate treatment and reducing mortality. Delayed diagnosis or inadequate therapy can lead to rapid disease progression and poor outcomes. Effective management strategies include:

- Prompt administration of antibiotics tailored to likely pathogens and local resistance patterns.
- Supportive care such as oxygen therapy, fluid resuscitation, and mechanical ventilation as needed.
- Adjunctive therapies like corticosteroids in select cases and antivirals for co-infections.

1.10 Conclusion

Severe community-acquired pneumonia remains a major public health challenge, with significant implications for individual patients and healthcare systems. Understanding its etiology, epidemiology, pathophysiology, and risk factors is essential for improving outcomes and guiding future research. Key areas for further investigation include the development of diagnostic biomarkers, pathogen-specific therapies, gene polymorphism, and strategies to reduce antimicrobial resistance. This chapter sets the stage for a comprehensive exploration of sCAP, delving into diagnostic approaches, therapeutic interventions, and preventive strategies in subsequent chapters.

References

1. Metlay JP, Waterer GW, Long AC, Anzueto A, Brozek J, Crothers K, et al. Diagnosis and treatment of adults with community-acquired pneumonia. *Am J Respir Crit Care Med.* 2019 October 1;200(7):E45–E67.
2. Lim WS, Van Der Eerden MM, Laing R, Boersma WG, Karalus N, Town GI, et al. Defining community acquired pneumonia severity on presentation to hospital: An international derivation and validation study [Internet]. *Thorax* 2003;58. Available from: www.thoraxjnl.com
3. Fine MJ, Auble TE, Yealy DM, Hanusa BH, Weissfeld LA, Singer DE, et al. A prediction rule to identify low-risk patients with community-acquired pneumonia. *N Engl J Med.* 1997;336(4):243–250.
4. Tsoumani E, Carter JA, Salomonsson S, Stephens JM, Bencina G. Clinical, economic, and humanistic burden of community acquired pneumonia in Europe: A systematic literature review. *Expert Rev Vaccines [Internet].* 2023 December 31;22(1):876–884. Available from: doi:10.1080/14760584.2023.2261785
5. Regunath H, Oba Y. Community-acquired pneumonia. In: *StatPearls* [Internet]. Updated 2024 January 26. Treasure Island (FL): StatPearls Publishing; 2024 [cited 2025 February 12]. Available from: https://www.ncbi.nlm.nih.gov/books/NBK430749/
6. Martin-Loeches I, Torres A, Nagavci B, Aliberti S, Antonelli M, Bassetti M, et al. ERS/ESICM/ESCMID/ALAT guidelines for the management of severe community-acquired pneumonia. *Intensive Care Med.* 2023 June 1;49(6):615–632.
7. Singh G, Widhani A, Shatri H, Sugiarto A, Aulia AN. Association between fraction and ratio of cd4/ cd8 bronchoalveolar lavage fluid toward extubation status and

mortality status of pneumonia severe patients in Dr. Cipto Mangunkusumo National General Hospital, Indonesia. *Indones J Chest* 2021;8(2):3–5.

8. Torres A, Cilloniz C, Niederman MS, Menéndez R, Chalmers JD, Wunderink RG, et al. Pneumonia. *Nat Rev Dis Primers [Internet]* 2021;7(1):25. Available from: doi:10.1038/s41572-021-00259-0

9. Apisarnthanarak A, Mundy LM. Etiology of community-acquired pneumonia. *Clin Chest Med.* W.B. Saunders; 2005;26(1):47–55.

10. Shoar S, Musher DM. Etiology of community-acquired pneumonia in adults: A systematic review. *Pneumonia* 2020 December;12(1):1–8.

11. Gadsby NJ, Musher DM. The microbial etiology of community-acquired pneumonia in adults: From classical bacteriology to host transcriptional signatures. *Clin Microbiol Rev* 2022;35: 3–5.

12. Niederman MS, Torres A. Severe community-acquired pneumonia. *Europ Resp Rev.* 2022 December 1;31(166): 3–5.

13. Salazar F, Bignell E, Brown GD, Cook PC, Warris A. Pathogenesis of respiratory viral and fungal coinfections 2021; Available from: doi:10.1128/CMR.00094-21

14. Cillóniz C, Ewig S, Ferrer M, Polverino E, Gabarrús A, Puig de la Bellacasa J, et al. Community-acquired polymicrobial pneumonia in the intensive care unit: Aetiology and prognosis. *Crit Care* 2011 September 14;15(5): 3–8.

15. Behar SM, Carpenter SM, Booty MG, Barber DL, Jayaraman P. Orchestration of pulmonary t cell immunity during mycobacterium tuberculosis infection: Immunity interruptus *Seminars Immunol.* Academic Press; 2014; 26(6):559–577.

16. Morgan AJ, Glossop AJ. Severe community-acquired pneumonia. *BJA Educ* 2016 May 1;16(5):167–172.

CHAPTER 2

Unraveling the Etiology and Achieving Accurate Diagnosis

2.1 Introduction

Bacterial pathogens are the primary etiological agents responsible for severe community-acquired pneumonia (sCAP), particularly in populations that are elderly, suffer from chronic diseases, or have compromised immune systems. Among these pathogens, *Streptococcus pneumoniae* remains the most frequently isolated organism. It is well known for its rapid onset, characterized by high fever, pleuritic chest pain, and rust-colored sputum. The bacterium's virulence is mainly attributed to its polysaccharide capsule, which facilitates immune evasion, and pneumolysin, a toxin that contributes to tissue damage. Increasingly, there are concerns regarding antibiotic resistance in *Streptococcus pneumoniae*, particularly in its ability to alter penicillin-binding proteins and macrolide efflux mechanisms (Figure 2.1).[1,2]

In addition to *Streptococcus pneumoniae*, other important pathogens implicated in sCAP include *Staphylococcus aureus*, especially methicillin-resistant *Staphylococcus*

DOI:10.1201/9781003629504-2

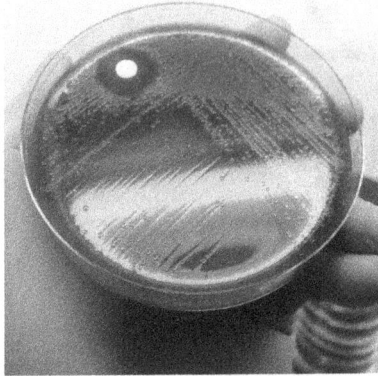

FIGURE 2.1 Gross colony morphology of *Streptococcus* on blood agar.

aureus (MRSA), which causes severe post-viral and necrotizing pneumonia. *Klebsiella pneumoniae*, a Gram-negative pathogen, is notably prevalent in patients with diabetes, chronic alcohol consumption, or those with recent hospitalizations. The bacterium is renowned for producing extended-spectrum beta-lactamases (ESBL) and carbapenemase enzymes, conferring resistance to many common antibiotics. *Escherichia coli*, traditionally associated with urinary tract and intra-abdominal infections, has also emerged as a significant cause of sCAP, especially in ICU patients or those with healthcare exposure. The increasing antimicrobial resistance observed in *Escherichia coli* complicates treatment strategies.[3,4]

Other pathogens, such as *Haemophilus influenzae* and *Moraxella catarrhalis*, are commonly implicated in exacerbations of chronic obstructive pulmonary disease (COPD) and pneumonia in older adults. These bacteria are often difficult to treat due to their ability to produce beta-lactamase enzymes. Additionally, Group A *Streptococcus* (GAS), well known for causing pharyngitis, can lead to severe toxin-mediated pneumonia in immunocompromised patients or during concurrent influenza outbreaks. Finally, anaerobic and microaerophilic organisms, such as *Peptostreptococcus* and *Fusobacterium*, are frequently found in aspiration pneumonia, especially in patients with swallowing difficulties or neurological impairments. These infections are typically polymicrobial and may present with foul-smelling sputum or cavitary disease.[1,2]

2.2 Etiology of Severe Community-Acquired Pneumonia

Pneumonia, particularly severe community-acquired pneumonia (sCAP), continues to represent a major global health concern due to its complex and multifactorial etiology. sCAP is associated with significant morbidity and mortality, especially among vulnerable populations such as the elderly, immunocompromised individuals, and those with underlying chronic conditions. In contrast to mild community-acquired pneumonia (CAP), sCAP typically involves highly virulent or multidrug-resistant organisms and is characterized by rapid clinical deterioration.

A comprehensive understanding of the diverse etiological agents responsible for sCAP, as well as the implementation of precise diagnostic strategies, is critical for timely treatment and improved patient outcomes. The pathogens that contribute to the development of sCAP encompass a wide range of microorganisms, including bacteria, viruses, fungi, and, less commonly, parasites. The prevalence of these causative agents is influenced by host-related factors, geographic variation, and evolving epidemiological trends. The subsequent sections will explore these causative microorganisms in greater detail.[2,3] The major pathogen groups implicated in sCAP, along with their clinical manifestations and risk profiles, are summarized in Tables 2.1 and 2.2.

TABLE 2.1 Summary of Pathogen Types in Severe Community-Acquired Pneumonia (sCAP)

Pathogen Type	Examples	Typical Clinical Features	Risk Groups
Bacterial	■ *Streptococcus pneumoniae* ■ *Staphylococcus aureus* (MRSA) ■ *Klebsiella pneumoniae* ■ *Escherichia coli* ■ *Haemophilus influenzae* ■ *Moraxella catarrhalis* ■ *Group A Streptococcus* ■ *Anaerobes (Peptostreptococcus, Fusobacterium)*	Acute onset fever, pleuritic chest pain, productive cough, cavitation (MRSA/Klebsiella), foul-smelling sputum (anaerobes)	Elderly, immunocompromised, COPD, diabetes, alcoholism
Atypical Bacteria	■ *Legionella pneumophila* ■ *Mycoplasma pneumoniae* ■ *Chlamydia pneumoniae* ■ *Coxiella burnetiid*	Dry cough, extrapulmonary symptoms (e.g., diarrhea, rash, hyponatremia), gradual onset	Young adults, closed communities (e.g., military, dormitories), livestock exposure
Viral	■ Influenza A/B ■ Respiratory syncytial virus (RSV) ■ Human metapneumovirus (hMPV) ■ Parainfluenza virus ■ Adenovirus ■ SARS-CoV-2	Fever, cough, myalgia, bilateral infiltrates, possible ARDS (especially SARS-CoV-2)	Elderly, immunocompromised, chronic illness

Category	Organisms	Clinical features	Epidemiology/risk factors
Fungal	■ Aspergillus fumigatus ■ Pneumocystis jirovecii ■ Cryptococcus spp. ■ Histoplasma capsulatum ■ Blastomyces dermatitidis ■ Coccidioides spp. ■ Mucorales (Rhizopus, Mucor)	Subacute or insidious symptoms, hypoxia, nodules or cavitation, bilateral ground-glass opacities, halo sign (Aspergillus), reversed halo sign (Mucorales)	HIV/AIDS, neutropenia, long-term steroids, transplant recipients
Parasitic	■ Toxoplasma gondii ■ Strongyloides stercoralis ■ Entamoeba histolytica ■ Paragonimus westermani ■ Schistosoma spp.	Fever, cough, diffuse infiltrates, eosinophilia (in some), hyperinfection syndrome (Strongyloides), hemoptysis or liver-pleural extension (Entamoeba)	Immunocompromised hosts, steroid users, HIV/AIDS, tropical or rural endemic exposure

TABLE 2.2 Key Bacterial Pathogens in Severe Community-Acquired Pneumonia

Pathogen	Characteristics/Associated Conditions	Clinical Presentation
Streptococcus pneumoniae	Most common, associated with advancing age, chronic diseases, immunocompromised states	Abrupt onset, high fever, pleuritic chest pain, rust-colored sputum
Staphylococcus aureus	Common post-viral, including influenza, COVID-19, and necrotizing pneumonia	Rapid progression, cavitary lesions, hemoptysis
Klebsiella pneumoniae	Prevalent in diabetics, chronic alcohol users, and recent hospitalizations	Lobar consolidation, "currant jelly" sputum
Escherichia coli	Associated with healthcare exposure, ICU patients, and increasing antimicrobial resistance	Fever, respiratory distress, difficulty in treatment due to resistance
Haemophilus influenzae	Common in COPD and older adults, contributing to exacerbations	Respiratory exacerbations, difficult to eradicate
Moraxella catarrhalis	Frequently implicated in COPD and exacerbations	Exacerbations, respiratory distress
Group A Streptococcus	Known for pharyngitis but can cause toxin-mediated pneumonia in immunocompromised patients	Severe pneumonia with systemic toxicity
Anaerobes (*Peptostreptococcus, Fusobacterium*)	Often involved in aspiration pneumonia, especially in those with swallowing difficulties	Cavitary disease, foul-smelling sputum

2.2.1 Bacteria

2.2.1.1 Streptococcus pneumoniae

Streptococcus pneumoniae is the most commonly identified bacterial cause of sCAP globally.[5] This Gram-positive, encapsulated diplococcus commonly colonizes the nasopharynx but can invade the lower respiratory tract in susceptible individuals, such as the elderly, those with chronic illnesses (e.g., COPD, heart failure), and immunocompromised hosts. Its key virulence factors include a polysaccharide capsule that inhibits phagocytosis, pneumolysin that disrupts epithelial integrity, and surface adhesins.[5]

Clinically, it presents with abrupt onset of fever, pleuritic chest pain, and productive cough, often with rust-colored sputum. Radiographic findings typically show lobar consolidation. Resistance has emerged particularly to penicillin and macrolides, driven by alterations in penicillin-binding proteins and efflux pump mechanisms.[6] Empiric therapy includes beta-lactams (e.g., ceftriaxone) plus a macrolide or fluoroquinolone.

2.2.1.2 Staphylococcus aureus

S. aureus, particularly MRSA, is a well-known cause of post-influenza and post-COVID-19 pneumonia.[7] It is a Gram-positive coccus in clusters and produces a range of virulence factors, including Panton-Valentine leukocidin (PVL), which can lead to necrotizing pneumonia with cavitary lesions, hemoptysis, and leukopenia.

MRSA strains show resistance to all beta-lactams via mecA gene-encoded altered PBP2a. Therapy often requires vancomycin or linezolid, with adjunctive clindamycin to inhibit toxin production in toxin-mediated disease.[8]

2.2.1.3 Klebsiella pneumoniae

K. pneumoniae is a Gram-negative, encapsulated bacillus that causes severe necrotizing pneumonia, particularly in alcoholics, diabetics, and hospitalized patients.[9] Its thick capsule contributes to mucoid colonies and protection from phagocytosis. Hallmark presentation includes high fever, productive cough with thick, blood-tinged "currant jelly" sputum, and lobar consolidation with bulging fissures on chest imaging.

Carbapenemase-producing strains are associated with extreme drug resistance. ESBL production limits the efficacy of many cephalosporins. Mortality rates can exceed 50% in immunocompromised patients.[10]

2.2.1.4 Escherichia coli

While primarily known for urosepsis and intra-abdominal infections, *E. coli* is an emerging sCAP pathogen, especially in patients with healthcare exposure, recent antibiotic use, or ICU admission.[11] It is a Gram-negative facultative anaerobe, and resistance to fluoroquinolones, third-generation cephalosporins, and carbapenems is rising.

Presentation can include fever, dyspnea, leukocytosis, and multilobar infiltrates. Given its resistance profile, empiric therapy often necessitates broad-spectrum agents such as carbapenems or cefepime.[12]

2.2.1.5 Haemophilus influenzae

H. influenzae is a small, Gram-negative coccobacillus, typically non-typeable strains in adults, and is especially relevant in COPD exacerbations and older adults with structural lung disease.[9,10] It can cause bronchopneumonia and often coexists with other pathogens.

Beta-lactamase production confers resistance to ampicillin and some cephalosporins. Treatment includes beta-lactam/beta-lactamase inhibitors or second-generation cephalosporins.

2.2.1.6 Moraxella catarrhalis

This Gram-negative diplococcus is a frequent colonizer of the upper respiratory tract but can cause lower respiratory infections in patients with COPD, asthma, or immunosuppression.[11] Like *H. influenzae*, it produces beta-lactamases, limiting the use of simple penicillins. Though typically less virulent, it can exacerbate chronic lung disease. It responds well to amoxicillin-clavulanate or macrolides.

2.2.1.7 Group A Streptococcus (GAS)

GAS (*S. pyogenes*) is an uncommon, but life-threatening cause of pneumonia, particularly in young, previously healthy adults during influenza epidemics.[12] Its exotoxins (SPE A, B, C) contribute to rapid progression to necrotizing pneumonia, sepsis, and streptococcal toxic shock syndrome.

Clinical suspicion is key; therapy includes high-dose beta-lactams and clindamycin for toxin suppression.

2.2.1.8 Anaerobes (e.g., Peptostreptococcus, Fusobacterium)

Anaerobes are implicated in aspiration pneumonia, lung abscesses, and necrotizing infections often in patients with altered consciousness, poor dentition, or swallowing disorders.[13] These are typically polymicrobial infections involving both anaerobes and aerobes.

Characteristic signs include foul-smelling sputum and cavitary lung lesions. Treatment involves clindamycin, ampicillin-sulbactam, or carbapenems.[14]

2.2.2 Atypical Bacteria

Atypical bacteria contribute to approximately 15–20% of community-acquired pneumonia cases and a significant subset of severe presentations (sCAP), especially in older adults, immunocompromised individuals, or those in crowded settings like nursing homes and military barracks.[15] These organisms differ from typical bacteria in several key aspects: many replicate intracellularly, lack a peptidoglycan-rich cell wall, and are unresponsive to beta-lactam antibiotics. They often present with extrapulmonary symptoms, complicating early diagnosis. Timely identification using molecular diagnostics and appropriate empiric coverage are crucial in suspected atypical infections.[16]

2.2.2.1 Legionella pneumophila

Legionella pneumophila is a Gram-negative, aerobic bacillus and the most clinically significant Legionella species. It thrives in artificial aquatic environments, such as air-conditioning systems, cooling towers, and plumbing. Human infection occurs via inhalation of aerosolized contaminated water.[17]

Once inhaled, *L. pneumophila* is phagocytosed by alveolar macrophages but evades destruction by preventing phagolysosomal fusion, leading to intracellular replication. It induces a robust inflammatory response, resulting in high fever, non-productive cough, gastrointestinal symptoms (e.g., diarrhea), hyponatremia, and altered mental status. Laboratory abnormalities may include elevated hepatic transaminases and C-reactive protein.

Standard culture is difficult, requiring buffered charcoal yeast extract (BCYE) agar. Rapid diagnosis is facilitated by urinary antigen testing (especially for serogroup 1) and Polymerase Chain Reaction (PCR).[18] Treatment relies on antibiotics with high intracellular penetration, such as fluoroquinolones (e.g., levofloxacin) or macrolides (e.g., azithromycin).

2.2.2.2 Mycoplasma pneumoniae

This organism lacks a cell wall, making it naturally resistant to beta-lactam antibiotics. It is transmitted via respiratory droplets and often affects children, adolescents, and young adults in school or military settings.[19]

Mycoplasma pneumoniae attaches to respiratory epithelium using P1 adhesin, causing cell injury through hydrogen peroxide and immune-mediated damage. The clinical course is typically insidious, with dry cough, low-grade fever, pharyngitis, and malaise. Extrapulmonary manifestations may include hemolytic anemia, rash, encephalitis, and myocarditis.[19]

Diagnosis is confirmed using PCR or IgM serology. First-line treatment is with macrolides; doxycycline or fluoroquinolones are alternatives in regions with high macrolide resistance or in adults.[19]

2.2.2.3 Chlamydia pneumoniae

C. pneumoniae is an obligate intracellular, Gram-negative bacterium that lacks a typical cell wall, rendering it unresponsive to beta-lactam agents.[20] It is spread via respiratory droplets and usually causes a slow-progressing lower respiratory tract infection.

Symptoms include sore throat, hoarseness, and dry cough. It is sometimes misdiagnosed as bronchitis or asthma due to its protracted course. Diagnosis relies on serology or PCR. Treatment options include macrolides, tetracyclines, or respiratory fluoroquinolones.[20]

2.2.2.4 Coxiella burnetii

C. burnetii, the causative agent of Q fever, is a spore-forming intracellular Gram-negative organism. Transmission typically occurs through inhalation of contaminated dust from infected livestock, posing an occupational risk to veterinarians, abattoir workers, and farmers.[21]

Acute Q fever presents with high fever, dry cough, fatigue, and hepatomegaly. Chest imaging may show segmental infiltrates. Chronic Q fever, more common in patients with valvular heart disease or immunosuppression, may progress to endocarditis.[21]

Diagnosis requires serologic testing for phase I and II antibodies or PCR. Acute cases are treated with doxycycline for 14 days, while chronic infections require prolonged therapy (e.g., doxycycline and hydroxychloroquine for ≥18 months).[22]

2.2.3 Viral Pathogens

Viral infections are increasingly recognized as significant contributors to sCAP, especially in vulnerable populations such as the elderly, immunocompromised individuals, and those with chronic cardiopulmonary comorbidities.[23] Viruses may act as primary pathogens or predispose patients to secondary bacterial infections through epithelial damage and immune dysregulation.

Recent studies report that respiratory viruses are detected in up to 30% of adults hospitalized with CAP, with seasonal variation and spikes during influenza epidemics or pandemics.[24] Accurate diagnosis requires the use of multiplex PCR panels due to the clinical overlap among viral and bacterial etiologies. While most viral pneumonias are self-limited, certain high-risk groups may develop respiratory failure requiring intensive care.

2.2.3.1 Influenza A and B

Influenza viruses remain the most frequently detected respiratory viruses in adult sCAP, particularly during winter epidemics. These segmented, negative-sense RNA viruses of the Orthomyxoviridae family cause sudden-onset fever, chills, myalgia, headache, and dry cough.[25] Primary viral pneumonia is a feared complication, especially in the elderly, pregnant women, and patients with underlying conditions such as heart failure or diabetes.

Radiologic findings typically include bilateral interstitial infiltrates, but may also show segmental consolidation. Early initiation of neuraminidase inhibitors (e.g., oseltamivir) within 48 hours of symptom onset has been shown to reduce morbidity and mortality.[26]

Coinfection with *Staphylococcus aureus*, *Streptococcus pneumoniae*, or MRSA is common and increases the risk of severe complications, including ARDS and septic shock.[27]

2.2.3.2 Respiratory Syncytial Virus (RSV)

Once considered primarily a pediatric pathogen, RSV is now increasingly recognized as a major cause of viral pneumonia in older adults, particularly those with COPD, heart failure, or immunosuppression.[28] Clinical features include fever, wheezing, dyspnea, and cough. Imaging may reveal interstitial infiltrates or peribronchial thickening.

Diagnosis is made via rapid antigen tests or PCR. Although specific antivirals for adults are limited, recent advances have led to the development of monoclonal antibodies and vaccines for older adults that reduce the risk of severe RSV disease.[29] Treatment remains supportive, including supplemental oxygen and, in severe cases, ventilatory support.

2.2.3.3 Human Metapneumovirus (hMPV)

hMPV is a paramyxovirus closely related to RSV and contributes to lower respiratory tract infections in the elderly and immunocompromised.[30] Symptoms include rhinorrhea, cough, and hypoxia. Like RSV, hMPV lacks targeted antiviral therapies, and treatment is largely supportive. Diagnosis is established through multiplex PCR testing of respiratory specimens.

2.2.3.4 SARS-CoV-2

SARS-CoV-2, the causative agent of COVID-19, has become the most prominent viral cause of sCAP since 2020. It presents with fever, cough, anosmia, and dyspnea, and may progress to ARDS in severe cases.[31] High-resolution chest CT often reveals bilateral ground-glass opacities with consolidation.

Management of severe COVID-19 includes antiviral agents (e.g., remdesivir), immunomodulators (e.g., corticosteroids, IL-6 inhibitors), and anticoagulation. Vaccination remains the most effective preventive measure.[32]

2.2.3.5 Other Viruses: Parainfluenza, Adenovirus, Non-SARS Coronaviruses

Parainfluenza viruses, adenovirus, and common human coronaviruses (OC43, 229E, NL63, HKU1) are less frequently associated with sCAP but can cause significant morbidity in older adults and immunocompromised patients.[33] Presentations are often indistinguishable from other viral pneumonias and include fever, sore throat, and cough. Diagnosis is primarily via multiplex PCR, and treatment is supportive.

Adenovirus pneumonia, though rare in adults, can be severe and necrotizing, particularly in transplant recipients or military recruits. It may present with hemoptysis and multi-organ dysfunction.

2.2.4 Fungal Pathogens

Fungal infections, though less prevalent than bacterial or viral causes, are increasingly implicated in sCAP, especially among patients with immunosuppression, hematologic malignancies, prolonged neutropenia, or recent corticosteroid use.[34] Prompt recognition is essential, as these infections can progress rapidly and require antifungal agents distinct from antibacterial therapies.

2.2.4.1 Aspergillus fumigatus

Aspergillus fumigatus is the most common cause of invasive pulmonary aspergillosis (IPA), particularly in individuals undergoing chemotherapy, hematopoietic stem cell or solid organ transplantation, and patients with influenza- or COVID-19-associated pulmonary injury.[35]

Clinically, IPA often presents with fever, dry cough, pleuritic chest pain, and hemoptysis. CT imaging may reveal nodular lesions with the characteristic "halo sign" in early stages or "air-crescent sign" during recovery.[36] As illustrated in Figure 2.2, a cavity was observed in the

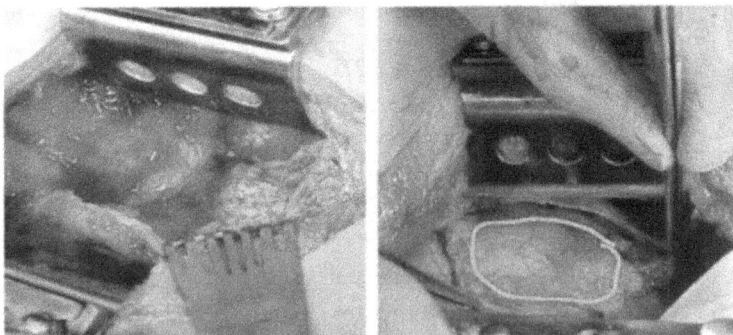

FIGURE 2.2 (Left) The cavity was found on the supeomedial lobe of the right lung. (Right) Granulomas were found disseminating the cavity (yellow circle).

superomedial lobe of the right lung (Left), with granulomas disseminating the cavity (yellow circle) (Right). Diagnosis requires a combination of clinical and radiologic suspicion along with laboratory confirmation, including galactomannan assay (serum or bronchoalveolar lavage), PCR, fungal culture, and histopathology showing acute-angle branching septate hyphae.[37]

First-line therapy includes voriconazole or isavuconazole; liposomal amphotericin B is reserved for cases of azole resistance or intolerance.[38]

2.2.4.2 Pneumocystis jirovecii

Pneumocystis jirovecii (formerly *P. carinii*) is a fungal organism that causes *Pneumocystis pneumonia* (PCP), predominantly in individuals with advanced HIV (CD4 <200 cells/μL), organ transplant recipients, and patients receiving high-dose corticosteroids.[39]

The clinical course is subacute, with progressive dyspnea, dry cough, and hypoxemia. Radiographic findings include diffuse bilateral ground-glass opacities. Serum β-D-glucan may aid in diagnosis, but definitive confirmation is obtained through PCR or immunofluorescence staining of BAL fluid.[40]

First-line treatment is high-dose trimethoprim-sulfamethoxazole (TMP-SMX), often accompanied by corticosteroids in patients with moderate-to-severe hypoxemia.[41]

2.2.4.3 Cryptococcus neoformans *and* C. gattii

These encapsulated yeasts primarily cause disease in individuals with HIV/AIDS, solid organ transplants, or corticosteroid use.[42] Pulmonary cryptococcosis may be asymptomatic or present with cough, chest pain, and fever; dissemination to the CNS can cause meningitis.

Imaging may show nodules, consolidation, or cavitary lesions. Diagnosis relies on serum and cerebrospinal fluid (CSF) cryptococcal antigen detection, fungal culture, and histopathology.[43] Treatment varies by disease severity and host immune status, often involving amphotericin B plus flucytosine followed by fluconazole.[44]

2.2.4.4 Histoplasma capsulatum

Histoplasma capsulatum is a dimorphic fungus endemic in the Ohio and Mississippi River valleys and parts of Southeast Asia. Infection occurs via inhalation of microconidia from environments contaminated by bird or bat droppings.[45]

Immunocompetent individuals may have mild or subclinical disease, while immunosuppressed hosts can develop disseminated histoplasmosis, presenting with fever, weight loss, hepatosplenomegaly, and diffuse pulmonary infiltrates. Diagnosis includes urine or serum antigen testing, fungal culture, and serology.[46]

Itraconazole is the preferred treatment for mild to moderate disease; severe cases may require liposomal amphotericin B followed by itraconazole.[47]

2.2.4.5 Blastomyces dermatitidis

This dimorphic fungus is found in North America, especially near the Great Lakes and river basins. Infection causes acute or chronic pneumonia and can disseminate to the skin, bone, or genitourinary tract.[48]

Symptoms include cough, fever, weight loss, and hemoptysis. Radiologically, it may resemble bacterial pneumonia or lung malignancy. Diagnosis requires culture or histopathology showing broad-based budding yeast.[49] Itraconazole is the mainstay of therapy; amphotericin B is used in severe disease.

2.2.4.6 Coccidioides immitis and C. posadasii

These fungi cause coccidioidomycosis ("Valley fever"), endemic in the southwestern U.S. and parts of Central/South America. Infection typically occurs via inhalation of arthroconidia from soil.[50]

While most cases are self-limited, high-risk individuals may develop severe pulmonary or disseminated disease. Symptoms include chest pain, cough, and fever. Imaging may reveal nodules, cavities, or hilar lymphadenopathy.

Diagnosis is based on serologic testing (IgM/IgG), fungal culture, or histopathology.[51]

Treatment includes fluconazole or itraconazole for mild disease; severe or disseminated cases may require amphotericin B.[52]

2.2.4.7 Mucormycosis

Mucormycosis is a rapidly progressive, angioinvasive fungal infection caused by *Mucorales* species, particularly *Rhizopus* and *Mucor*. It affects patients with uncontrolled diabetes, diabetic ketoacidosis, hematologic malignancies, or prolonged corticosteroid use.[53]

Pulmonary mucormycosis may manifest with fever, hemoptysis, and pleuritic pain. Imaging may show infarcts, cavitation, or the reversed halo sign. Diagnosis relies on histopathologic identification of broad, ribbon-like, non-septate hyphae with right-angle branching, and fungal culture or PCR.[54]

Management includes urgent surgical debridement and antifungal therapy with high-dose liposomal amphotericin B or isavuconazole.[55]

2.2.5 Parasitic Pathogens

Although uncommon, parasitic infections can cause severe community-acquired pneumonia (sCAP), particularly in immunocompromised individuals, those from or traveling to endemic regions, and patients receiving long-term corticosteroids or cytotoxic therapy.[56] Parasitic pulmonary infections may manifest as diffuse alveolar infiltrates, eosinophilic pneumonia, or hemorrhagic pneumonitis, and are frequently underdiagnosed due to non-specific presentation and limited diagnostic suspicion.

2.2.5.1 Toxoplasma gondii

Toxoplasma gondii is an obligate intracellular protozoan most commonly associated with encephalitis in patients with AIDS (CD4 <100 cells/μL). However, pulmonary toxoplasmosis may also occur, particularly in patients with profound immunosuppression such as hematologic malignancies or organ transplantation.[57]

Clinical manifestations include dyspnea, fever, and non-productive cough, often mimicking *Pneumocystis jirovecii* pneumonia. Radiologic findings show bilateral interstitial or alveolar infiltrates. Diagnosis is confirmed through PCR detection in bronchoalveolar lavage (BAL) fluid, serology (IgG/IgM), or histopathology.[58] Treatment typically involves high-dose pyrimethamine, sulfadiazine, and leucovorin.[59]

2.2.5.2 Strongyloides stercoralis

Strongyloides stercoralis is a soil-transmitted helminth endemic in tropical and subtropical regions. It is capable of causing life-threatening hyperinfection syndrome in immunocompromised hosts, particularly those receiving corticosteroids, transplant recipients, and patients with HTLV-1 infection.[60]

Pulmonary involvement includes wheezing, dyspnea, cough, and diffuse alveolar hemorrhage. Dissemination of larvae through the lungs may cause Gram-negative bacteremia and sepsis. Radiological features include bilateral infiltrates or alveolar hemorrhage.

Diagnosis is established by identifying larvae in sputum, BAL fluid, or stool, and eosinophilia may be absent in hyperinfection. PCR and serologic assays may assist diagnosis.[61] Ivermectin is the treatment of choice, and early administration is critical for survival.[62]

2.2.5.3 Entamoeba histolytica

While *Entamoeba histolytica* primarily causes intestinal amebiasis and liver abscesses, pulmonary involvement can result from rupture of an amebic liver abscess into the pleural space or lung parenchyma.[63]

Patients may present with fever, cough, right upper quadrant pain, and purulent or anchovy-paste-like sputum. Diagnosis is supported by imaging showing subdiaphragmatic abscess and pleuropulmonary extension, along with serologic testing.[64]

Treatment involves metronidazole to eliminate tissue trophozoites followed by a luminal agent (e.g., paromomycin) to eradicate intestinal colonization.[65]

2.2.5.4 Paragonimus westermani

Paragonimus westermani, also known as the oriental lung fluke, is endemic to parts of East and Southeast Asia and is acquired through ingestion of undercooked freshwater crustaceans. After translocation from the intestine to the lungs, the parasite causes chronic eosinophilic pneumonia.[66]

Clinical features include chronic cough, hemoptysis, chest pain, and eosinophilia. Radiologic findings often mimic tuberculosis, showing cavitary lesions or nodules. Diagnosis is made by identifying ova in sputum, BAL fluid, or stool, and serologic testing.[67] Treatment is with praziquantel for 2–3 days.[68]

2.2.5.5 Schistosoma spp.

Pulmonary involvement in *Schistosoma* infection may lead to pulmonary hypertension due to chronic egg embolization and granulomatous inflammation in the pulmonary vasculature.[69] Patients typically have a history of freshwater exposure in endemic regions. Symptoms include dyspnea on exertion and signs of right heart strain. Diagnosis is based on serology, stool/urine microscopy for ova, and echocardiographic findings of pulmonary hypertension. Praziquantel remains the mainstay of treatment, but pulmonary vascular changes may be irreversible in late-stage disease.[70]

2.3 Conclusion

The etiology of severe community-acquired pneumonia (sCAP) is diverse, encompassing typical and atypical bacteria, respiratory viruses, fungi, and occasionally parasites, particularly in immunocompromised populations.

While *Streptococcus pneumoniae* and *Legionella pneumophila* remain leading bacterial causes, emerging pathogens such as influenza, RSV, SARS-CoV-2, and fungal species like *Aspergillus* and *Pneumocystis jirovecii* are increasingly recognized as major contributors to morbidity and mortality. Accurate identification of the causative agent is essential for timely and targeted therapy, as well as for implementing appropriate infection control strategies. A thorough understanding of the patient's risk factors, geographic exposure, and immune status is crucial for guiding the diagnostic approach. Integration of conventional microbiological methods with rapid diagnostics and biomarkers enhances the ability to tailor treatment and improve clinical outcomes in sCAP.

References

1. Lim WS, Baudouin SV, George RC, et al. BTS guidelines for the management of community acquired pneumonia in adults. *Thorax.* 2009;64(Suppl 3):iii1–iii55.
2. Claessens YE, Debray MP, Tubach F, et al. Early chest CT scan to assist diagnosis and guide treatment decision for suspected community-acquired pneumonia. *Am J Respir Crit Care Med.* 2015;192(8):974–982.
3. Metlay JP, Waterer GW, Long AC, et al. Diagnosis and treatment of adults with community-acquired pneumonia: An official clinical practice guideline of the American Thoracic Society and Infectious Diseases Society of America. *Am J Respir Crit Care Med.* 2019;200(7):e45–e67.
4. Schuetz P, Wirz Y, Sager R, et al. Procalcitonin to initiate or discontinue antibiotics in acute respiratory tract infections. *Cochrane Database Syst Rev.* 2017;10(10):CD007498.
5. Feldman C, Anderson R. Recent advances in the epidemiology and prevention of Streptococcus pneumoniae infections. *F1000Res.* 2020;9:F1000 Faculty Rev-338.
6. Lynch JP, Zhanel GG. Streptococcus pneumoniae: Epidemiology and risk factors, evolution of antimicrobial resistance, and impact of vaccines. *Curr Opin Pulm Med.* 2010;16(3):217–225.

7. Tong SY, Davis JS, Eichenberger E, Holland TL, Fowler VG Jr. Staphylococcus aureus infections: Epidemiology, pathophysiology, clinical manifestations, and management. *Clin Microbiol Rev.* 2015;28(3):603–661.

8. Kollef MH, Micek ST. Methicillin-resistant Staphylococcus aureus: A new community-acquired pathogen? *Curr Opin Infect Dis.* 2006;19(2):123–127.

9. Podschun R, Ullmann U. Klebsiella spp. as nosocomial pathogens: Epidemiology, taxonomy, typing methods, and pathogenicity factors. *Clin Microbiol Rev.* 1998;11(4):589–603.

10. Pitout JD, Laupland KB. Extended-spectrum β-lactamase-producing *Enterobacteriaceae*: An emerging public-health concern. *Lancet Infect Dis.* 2008;8(3):159–166.

11. Sader HS, Farrell DJ, Flamm RK, Jones RN. Antimicrobial susceptibility of *Haemophilus influenzae* and *Moraxella catarrhalis* collected in the United States and Europe during 2010–2011. *Antimicrob Agents Chemother.* 2014; 58(4):2241–2245.

12. Musher DM. Clinical and microbiological end points in the treatment of pneumonia. *Clin Infect Dis.* 2008;47(Suppl 3):S207–S209.

13. Marik PE. Aspiration pneumonitis and aspiration pneumonia. *N Engl J Med.* 2001;344(9):665–671.

14. Bartlett JG. Anaerobic bacterial infections of the lung and pleural space. *Clin Infect Dis.* 1993;16(Suppl 4):S248–S255.

15. Jain S, et al. Community-acquired pneumonia requiring hospitalization among U.S. adults. *N Engl J Med.* 2015;373(5):415–427.

16. Mandell LA, et al. Infectious diseases society of America/ American thoracic society consensus guidelines on the management of CAP in adults. *Clin Infect Dis.* 2007;44 Suppl 2:S27–S72.

17. Diederen BMW. *Legionella* spp. and Legionnaires' disease. *J Infect.* 2008;56(1):1–12.

18. Phin N, et al. Epidemiology and clinical management of Legionnaires' disease. *Lancet Infect Dis.* 2014;14(10): 1011–1021.

19. Waites KB, et al. Mycoplasma pneumoniae from the respiratory tract and beyond. *Clin Microbiol Rev.* 2017; 30(3):747–809.

20. Hahn DL. *Chlamydia pneumoniae*, asthma, and COPD: What is the evidence? *Ann Allergy Asthma Immunol.* 1999;83(4):271–292.

21. Raoult D, Marrie T, Mege J-L. Natural history and pathophysiology of Q fever. *Lancet Infect Dis.* 2005;5(4):219–226.

22. Anderson A, et al. Diagnosis and management of Q fever: United States, 2013. *MMWR Recomm Rep.* 2013;62(RR-03):1–30.

23. Falsey AR, et al. Viral pneumonia in older adults. *Clin Infect Dis.* 2005;40(4):521–528.

24. Jain S, et al. Community-acquired pneumonia requiring hospitalization among U.S. adults. *N Engl J Med.* 2015;373(5):415–427.

25. Uyeki TM. Influenza. *Ann Intern Med.* 2022; 175(1):ITC1–ITC16.

26. Muthuri SG, et al. Effectiveness of neuraminidase inhibitors in reducing mortality in patients hospitalized with influenza A(H1N1)pdm09 virus infection. *Lancet Respir Med.* 2014;2(5):395–404.

27. Morris DE, et al. Secondary bacterial infections associated with influenza pandemics. *Front Microbiol.* 2017;8:1041.

28. Ackerson B, et al. Severe respiratory syncytial virus infection in adults. *Clin Infect Dis.* 2019;69(6):1118–1124.

29. Walsh EE, et al. A bivalent RSV prefusion F vaccine in older adults. *N Engl J Med.* 2023;388(7):595–608.

30. Boivin G, et al. Human metapneumovirus infections in hospitalized adults. *Emerg Infect Dis.* 2003;9(10): 1263–1266.

31. Guan WJ, et al. Clinical characteristics of coronavirus disease 2019 in China. *N Engl J Med.* 2020;382(18): 1708–1720.

32. Recovery Collaborative Group. Dexamethasone in hospitalized patients with Covid-19. *N Engl J Med.* 2021;384(8):693–704.

33. Templeton KE, et al. Comparison and evaluation of real-time PCR, shell vial culture, and conventional cell culture for the detection of respiratory viruses. *J Med Virol.* 2004;72(3): 304–313.

34. Marr KA, et al. Fungal infection in acute respiratory illness. *Clin Chest Med.* 2009;30(2):409–426.

35. Schauwvlieghe AFAD, et al. Invasive aspergillosis in influenza patients in the ICU. *Am J Respir Crit Care Med.* 2018;198(4):520–522.

36. Kousha M, et al. Pulmonary aspergillosis: a clinical review. *Eur Respir Rev.* 2011;20(121):156–174.
37. Patterson TF, et al. Practice guidelines for the diagnosis and management of aspergillosis. *Clin Infect Dis.* 2016;63(4):e1–e60.
38. Herbrecht R, et al. Voriconazole versus amphotericin B for invasive aspergillosis. *N Engl J Med.* 2002;347(6):408–415.
39. Yale SH, Limper AH. *Pneumocystis carinii* pneumonia in patients without AIDS: associated illnesses and prior corticosteroid therapy. *Mayo Clin Proc.* 1996;71(1):5–13.
40. Alanio A, et al. Real-time PCR assay for diagnosis of *Pneumocystis jirovecii* pneumonia. *J Clin Microbiol.* 2011;49(2):704–709.
41. Thomas CF, Limper AH. Pneumocystis pneumonia. *N Engl J Med.* 2004;350(24):2487–2498.
42. Park BJ, et al. Estimation of the current global burden of cryptococcal meningitis among persons living with HIV/AIDS. *AIDS.* 2009;23(4):525–530.
43. Perfect JR, et al. Clinical practice guidelines for cryptococcal disease. *Clin Infect Dis.* 2010;50(3):291–322.
44. Jarvis JN, Harrison TS. Pulmonary cryptococcosis. *Semin Respir Crit Care Med.* 2008;29(2):141–150.
45. Kauffman CA. Histoplasmosis. *Clin Chest Med.* 2009; 30(2):217–225.
46. Hage CA, et al. Histoplasmosis: up-to-date evidence-based approach to diagnosis and management. *Semin Respir Crit Care Med.* 2015;36(5):729–745.
47. Wheat LJ, et al. Clinical practice guidelines for the management of patients with histoplasmosis. *Clin Infect Dis.* 2007;45(7):807–825.
48. Saccente M, Woods GL. Clinical and laboratory update on blastomycosis. *Clin Microbiol Rev.* 2010;23(2): 367–381.
49. Smith JA, Kauffman CA. Blastomycosis. *Proc Am Thorac Soc.* 2010;7(3):173–180.
50. Galgiani JN, et al. Coccidioidomycosis. *Clin Infect Dis.* 2005;41(9):1217–1223.
51. Ampel NM. Coccidioidomycosis in persons infected with HIV type 1. *Clin Infect Dis.* 2005;41(8):1174–1178.
52. Johnson RH, et al. Coccidioidomycosis: A review. *JAMA.* 2021;326(13):1242–1252.

53. Roden MM, et al. Epidemiology and outcome of zygomycosis: A review of 929 reported cases. *Clin Infect Dis.* 2005;41(5):634–653.
54. Spellberg B, et al. Mucormycosis: Pathogenesis, clinical manifestations, and therapy. *Clin Infect Dis.* 2005;41(5): 634–653.
55. Cornely OA, et al. Global guideline for the diagnosis and management of mucormycosis. *Lancet Infect Dis.* 2019;19(12):e405–e421.
56. Martinez-Giron R, et al. Parasitic pulmonary infections in immunocompromised patients. *Respiration.* 2015;89(4):253–262.
57. Derouin F, Pelloux H. Prevention of toxoplasmosis in transplant patients. *Clin Microbiol Infect.* 2008; 14(12):1089–1101.
58. Robert-Gangneux F, Dardé ML. Epidemiology of and diagnostic strategies for toxoplasmosis. *Clin Microbiol Rev.* 2012;25(2):264–296.
59. Montoya JG, Liesenfeld O. Toxoplasmosis. *Lancet.* 2004;363(9425):1965–1976.
60. Keiser PB, Nutman TB. *Strongyloides stercoralis* in the immunocompromised population. *Clin Microbiol Rev.* 2004;17(1):208–217.
61. Buonfrate D, et al. *Strongyloides stercoralis*: the need for accurate diagnosis. *PLoS Negl Trop Dis.* 2020;14(10):e0008220.
62. Mejia R, Nutman TB. Screening, prevention, and treatment for hyperinfection syndrome due to *Strongyloides stercoralis*. *Curr Opin Infect Dis.* 2012;25(4):458–463.
63. Reed SL. Amebiasis: An update. *Clin Infect Dis.* 1992; 14(2):385–393.
64. Sharma MP, Ahuja V. Amoebic liver abscess. *J Indian Acad Clin Med.* 2003;4(2):107–111.
65. Blessmann J, et al. Comparison of nitroimidazoles for treatment of amoebiasis. *Trans R Soc Trop Med Hyg.* 2003;97(4):443–446.
66. Singh TS, Sugiyama H, Rangsiruji A. *Paragonimus* and paragonimiasis in India. *Indian J Med Res.* 2012;136(2): 192–204.
67. Nakamura-Uchiyama F, et al. Paragonimiasis: A Japanese perspective. *Clin Chest Med.* 2002;23(2):409–420.

68. Blair D, et al. Paragonimiasis and the genus *Paragonimus*. *Adv Parasitol*. 1999;42:113–222.
69. Ferreira RM, et al. Schistosomiasis and pulmonary arterial hypertension: Update on pathophysiology and treatment. *Curr Opin Pulm Med*. 2021;27(5):353–360.
70. Andrade ZA. Schistosomiasis and liver fibrosis. *Parasite Immunol*. 2009;31(11):656–663.

CHAPTER 3

Imaging Etiology of Pneumonia

3.1 Introduction

Pneumonia remains a leading cause of morbidity and mortality worldwide, particularly among vulnerable populations such as the elderly, the immunocompromised, and those with chronic health conditions. While clinical symptoms such as fever, cough, dyspnea, and pleuritic chest pain form the cornerstone of suspicion, imaging plays an indispensable role in the diagnosis, classification, and management of this complex disease. Understanding the various imaging manifestations of pneumonia not only allows for accurate diagnosis but also guides therapeutic decision-making and prognostication.[1]

3.2 Imaging Modalities in Pneumonia

Radiographic imaging, particularly chest radiography, is often the first-line modality in evaluating suspected pneumonia. Its accessibility and cost-effectiveness make it a ubiquitous diagnostic tool in both outpatient and inpatient settings. The detection of new pulmonary opacities on chest X-ray, in the context of compatible clinical

 DOI:10.1201/9781003629504-3

findings, fulfills the diagnostic criteria for pneumonia. Nevertheless, radiography may be limited by its inability to detect early or subtle disease, especially in immuno-compromised patients or those with minimal symptoms. In such cases, computed tomography (CT) becomes indispensable, providing high-resolution images that unveil parenchymal changes otherwise obscured on plain radiographs.[2]

CT imaging allows for detailed evaluation of lung architecture and pathology, enabling the identification of ground-glass opacities, cavitation, bronchial wall thickening, and nodular patterns. These findings often correspond with specific infectious pathogens and pathophysiologic processes. Moreover, CT is pivotal in recognizing complications such as empyema, abscess formation, necrotizing pneumonia, and bronchopleural fistulas.[2-3]

3.3 Imaging Patterns According to Etiology

The imaging appearance of pneumonia varies considerably depending on the etiologic agent, host immune status, and the presence of comorbidities. Traditionally, three classical patterns have been described: lobar or segmental pneumonia, bronchopneumonia, and atypical pneumonia.[3-4]

3.3.1 Lobar or Segmental Pneumonia

Lobar pneumonia typically presents with homogeneous consolidation involving a lung segment or entire lobe. The classical radiologic sign associated with this pattern is the air bronchogram, reflecting aerated bronchi surrounded by consolidated alveoli. *Streptococcus pneumoniae* is the archetypal pathogen causing this pattern. Other organisms, such as *Legionella, Haemophilus influenzae,* and *Klebsiella pneumoniae,* may produce similar findings, with *Klebsiella* sometimes showing the "bulging fissure sign" due to expansive consolidation (Figure 3.1).[3-4]

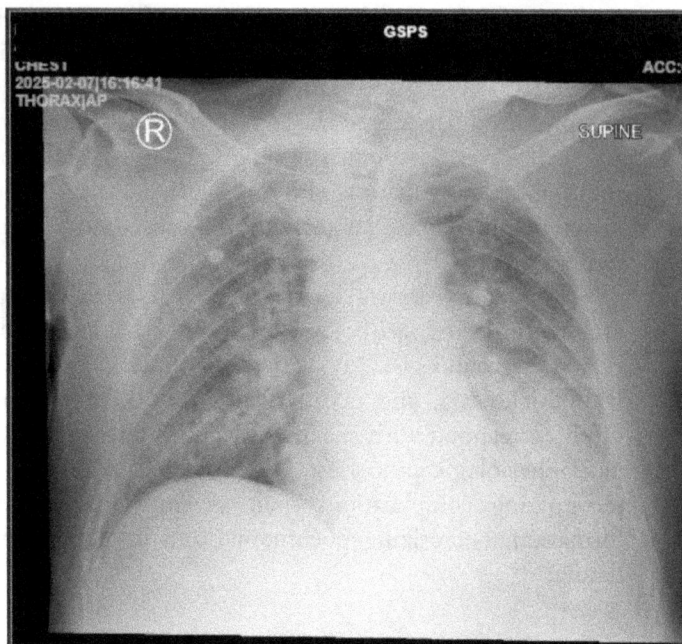

FIGURE 3.1 Chest radiograph (PA view) and axial CT scan demonstrating right upper lobe consolidation with air bronchograms in a patient with *Streptococcus pneumoniae* pneumonia.

3.3.2 Bronchopneumonia

Bronchopneumonia is characterized by patchy, multifocal consolidation centered around bronchi and bronchioles. On CT, this manifests as peribronchovascular and centrilobular nodules, sometimes forming the tree-in-bud pattern. This pattern is often seen with bacterial pathogens such as *Staphylococcus aureus* and *Pseudomonas aeruginosa*, particularly in nosocomial infections. Complications including cavitation and pleural effusions are common.[2–3]

3.3.3 Atypical Pneumonia

Atypical pneumonia includes infections caused by pathogens such as *Mycoplasma pneumoniae*, respiratory viruses including Influenza A, and certain fungi. The

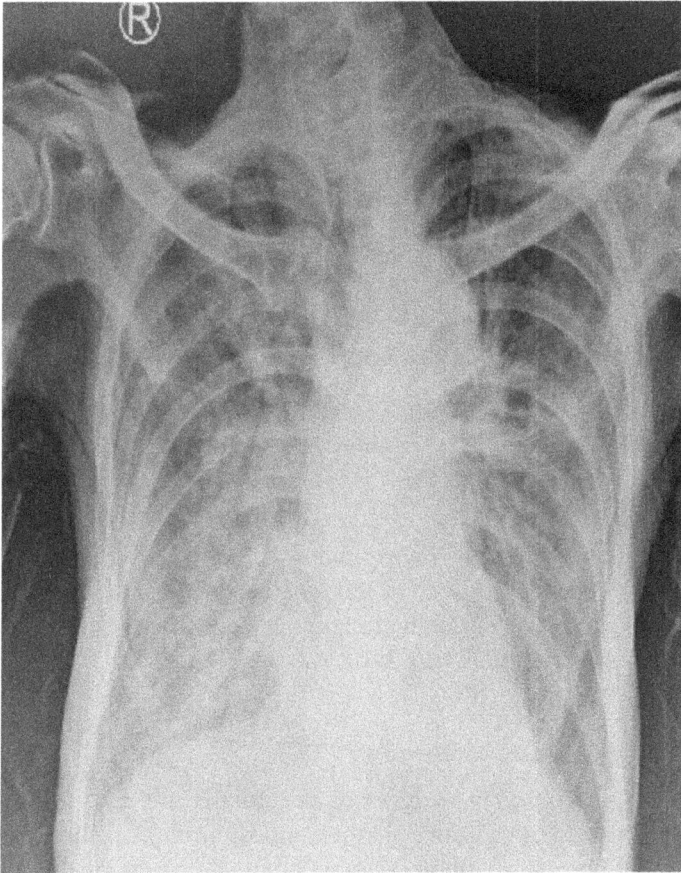

FIGURE 3.2 Chest radiograph showing bilateral patchy infiltrates and reticular opacities, consistent with atypical pneumonia.

imaging findings are generally more subtle, often involving ground-glass opacities, reticular patterns, and small nodules (Figure 3.2).[5]

3.3.4 Special Imaging Features

3.3.4.1 Halo Sign in Angioinvasive Fungal Infection

In immunocompromised patients, angioinvasive fungal infections, especially due to *Aspergillus* species, may demonstrate the halo sign on CT imaging, a nodular or

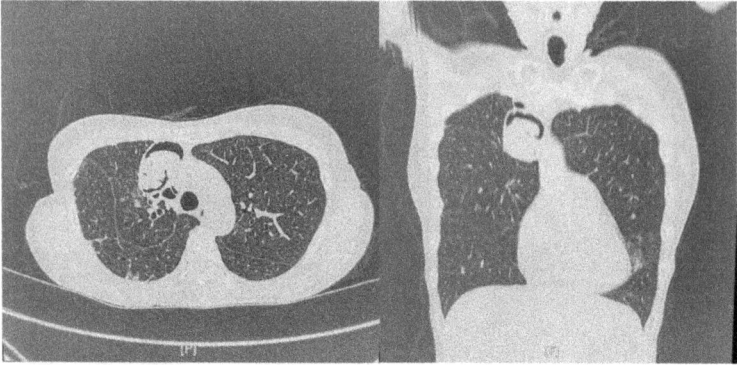

FIGURE 3.3 Axial chest CT showing cavitary lesion with surrounding ground-glass halo in a patient with invasive pulmonary aspergillosis.

mass-like lesion surrounded by a ground-glass opacity halo. This finding indicates hemorrhagic infarction due to vascular invasion by fungal hyphae and is a critical diagnostic clue (Figure 3.3).[6]

3.4 Conclusion

The imaging patterns of pneumonia are diverse, influenced by causative organisms, host immunity, and disease severity. Radiologists play a crucial role in synthesizing imaging with clinical and laboratory data for accurate diagnosis. This chapter highlights key imaging features for common pathogens, including *Streptococcus pneumoniae*, Influenza A virus, and *Aspergillus* species, illustrated by selected radiographic and CT images. Understanding these imaging hallmarks remains essential in guiding effective management amid the challenges posed by emerging pathogens and antimicrobial resistance.

References

1. Walker CM, Abbott GF, Greene RE, et al. Imaging pulmonary infection: classic signs and patterns. *AJR Am J Roentgenol.* 2014;202(4):674–684.
2. Franquet T. *Imaging of Pulmonary Infection.* Springer; 2019.
3. Cook AE, Garrana SH, Martínez-Jiménez S, Rosado-de-Christenson ML. Imaging Patterns of Pneumonia. *Semin Roentgenol.* 2021;57(1):18–29.
4. Franquet T. Imaging of community-acquired pneumonia. *J Thorac Imaging.* 2018;33(5):282–294.
5. Koo HJ, Lim S, Choe J, et al. Radiographic and CT features of viral pneumonia. *Radiographics.* 2018;38(3):719–739.
6. Kanne JP, Yandow DR, Meyer CA. Pneumocystis jiroveci pneumonia: high-resolution CT findings in patients with and without HIV infection. *AJR Am J Roentgenol.* 2012;198(3):W555–W561.

CHAPTER 4

Unravelling the Immunology of Host Response

4.1 Introduction

Severe community-acquired pneumonia (sCAP) results from an intricate balance between pathogen virulence and host immune response. While pathogen elimination is critical, evidence suggests that either an excessive inflammatory response or subsequent immune suppression can significantly impact disease progression and mortality. A better understanding of these immunological processes is key to developing new therapeutic approaches aimed at immune modulation.[1]

4.2 Local Immunopathology in Severe Community-Acquired Pneumonia

In sCAP, local immune dysregulation significantly influences the extent of lung injury and clinical outcomes. Alveolar macrophages are pivotal in host defense, facilitating pathogen clearance and modulating inflammatory responses. However, hyperactivation of these macrophages, indicated by elevated levels of soluble triggering

DOI:10.1201/9781003629504-4

receptor expressed on myeloid cells (sTREM-1), can provoke an excessive inflammatory cascade.[1]

The release of interleukin-6 (IL-6) by alveolar macrophages further amplifies inflammation by promoting the differentiation of CD4+ T cells into Th17 cells, contributing to heightened immune activation.[2,3] Moreover, regulatory T cells expressing the transcription factor Foxp3 support epithelial repair mechanisms by enhancing surfactant protein A (SP-A) production, which is crucial for maintaining alveolar homeostasis.[4-6]

Low CD4+ T-cell counts in bronchoalveolar lavage fluid (BALF) have been linked to poor extubation outcomes and higher mortality rates, emphasizing the protective role of local adaptive immunity.[7] Dysregulation of this balance, particularly via unregulated alveolar macrophage apoptosis mediated by caspase-3, may impair pathogen clearance and accelerate lung injury progression.[3]

A recent prospective cohort study demonstrated that low alveolar macrophage function, reduced BALF IL-6 levels, and elevated BALF CD4+ cell counts were significantly associated with successful extubation and improved survival in patients with severe pneumonia (Figure 4.1).[7]

Besides the well-described functions of alveolar macrophages and CD4+ T cells, recent insights suggest that monocyte-derived macrophages (Mo-Macs) may also infiltrate the alveolar spaces during severe pneumonia and contribute to dysregulated inflammation. These cells are typically recruited from circulation in response to chemokines such as MCP-1 and may differ functionally from resident alveolar macrophages, displaying higher pro-inflammatory potential.[8] Furthermore, dendritic cells residing in the lung mucosa not only prime T-cell responses but also influence tolerance mechanisms; their dysfunction in sCAP could tip the immune balance toward unregulated inflammation.[9]

In addition, epithelial cells are not merely passive barriers but active participants in immune signaling. They produce antimicrobial peptides like defensins and

SEVERELY AFFECTED LUNG

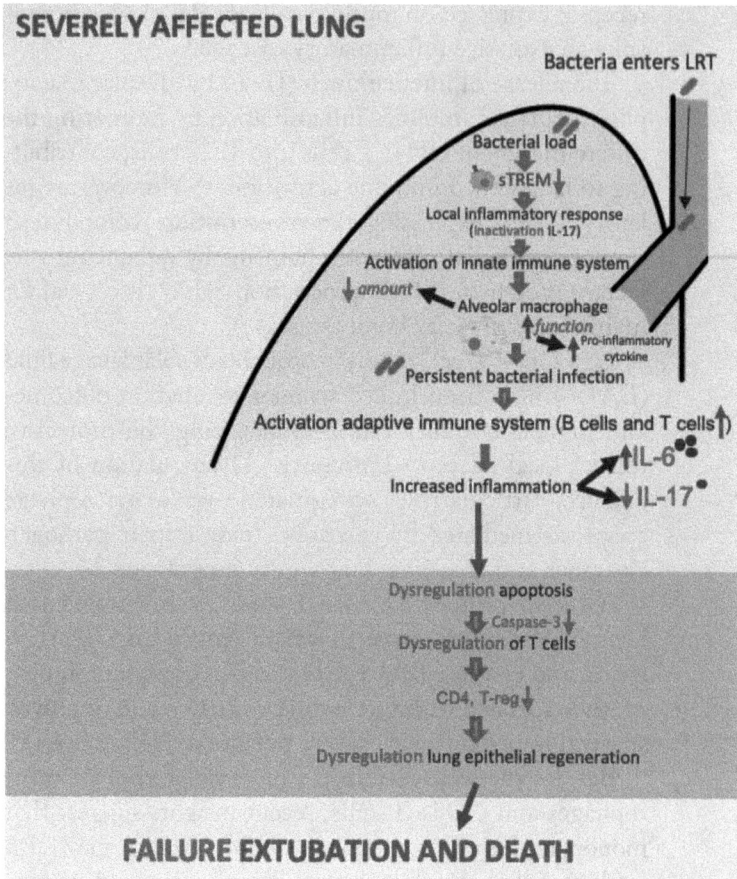

Bacteria enters LRT

Bacterial load

sTREM↓

Local inflammatory response
(Inactivation IL-17)

Activation of innate immune system

↓*amount*

Alveolar macrophage

↑*function*

Pro-inflammatory
cytokine

Persistent bacterial infection

Activation adaptive immune system (B cells and T cells↑)

Increased inflammation

↑IL-6

↓IL-17

Dysregulation apoptosis

Caspase-3

Dysregulation of T cells

CD4, T-reg↓

Dysregulation lung epithelial regeneration

FAILURE EXTUBATION AND DEATH

FIGURE 4.1 Pathophysiology of local immunopathology in severe lung injury injury (extubation failure and death).[7]

cathelicidins, and contribute to immune cell recruitment via chemokines such as CXCL8. Loss of epithelial integrity due to inflammation or pathogen-mediated cytotoxicity (e.g., pneumolysin) exposes underlying tissue to secondary insults and perpetuates the inflammatory cycle.[6,10]

4.2.1 The Role of the Innate Immune System

The innate immune system forms the body's initial defense against invading pathogens. Pattern recognition receptors (PRRs) such as toll-like receptors (TLRs) and NOD-like receptors (NLRs) recognize microbial structures and activate inflammatory cascades that release cytokines, including IL-1β, IL-6, and TNF-α. These mediators attract neutrophils and macrophages to the infection site, aiding pathogen clearance. However, in sCAP, excessive neutrophil activity and the formation of neutrophil extracellular traps (NETs) may lead to endothelial damage and exacerbate lung injury, contributing to respiratory failure and systemic complications.[3,7]

Beyond neutrophils and macrophages, natural killer (NK) cells are increasingly recognized as early effectors in pneumonia. They exert cytotoxic effects against infected cells and release IFN-γ, amplifying macrophage activity. However, dysregulation or exhaustion of NK cells, marked by overexpression of NKG2A, has been documented in critical illness, correlating with poor outcomes in pneumonia.[11]

Moreover, recent studies highlight the contribution of innate lymphoid cells (ILCs), particularly group 3 ILCs, in producing IL-22, a cytokine essential for epithelial barrier repair. Reduced IL-22 levels have been associated with worsened epithelial injury and higher bacterial load in experimental pneumonia models.[12]

4.2.2 The Adaptive Immune Response

The adaptive immune system is activated through antigen presentation by dendritic cells and macrophages, which stimulate T and B lymphocytes. CD4+ T-helper cells play a pivotal role in orchestrating pathogen defense, with Th1 and Th17 subsets particularly significant. Nevertheless, excessive Th17 responses can intensify lung inflammation and tissue injury. Furthermore, B cells are essential for antibody production, including the generation of immunoglobulin G (IgG) and immunoglobulin M (IgM), which are crucial for pathogen neutralization and clearance. Inadequate humoral immunity, marked by impaired antibody responses, is associated with poor clinical outcomes in sCAP patients.[2,7]

Beyond CD4+ T-cell subsets, CD8+ cytotoxic T lymphocytes (CTLs) play a role in eliminating virus-infected and some bacterial-infected cells via perforin and granzyme pathways. However, in the context of sCAP, their activation may also contribute to collateral tissue damage, especially in viral–bacterial coinfections such as influenza complicated by *Streptococcus pneumoniae*.[13]

Emerging evidence also underscores the role of T follicular helper (Tfh) cells in orchestrating germinal center reactions and promoting high-affinity antibody production. Impaired Tfh function in critical illness has been linked to suboptimal B-cell responses and reduced class switch recombination.[14]

4.2.3 Immunosuppression Following Hyperinflammation

After an intense initial inflammatory response, patients with sCAP may develop an immunosuppressive phase known as immunoparalysis. This is characterized by T-cell exhaustion, diminished antigen presentation capacity, and upregulation of inhibitory receptors such as PD-1 and CTLA-4. This state increases vulnerability to secondary infections, which may worsen disease outcomes.[3]

In addition to PD-1 and CTLA-4, other immune checkpoints, such as TIM-3 and LAG-3, are also implicated in post-inflammatory immune exhaustion. These receptors suppress T-cell effector function and are often co-expressed on exhausted T cells, especially in prolonged ICU stays.[15] Importantly, this state is also marked by myeloid-derived suppressor cells (MDSCs) expansion, which dampens antigen presentation and T-cell activation, contributing to prolonged immunosuppression and nosocomial infection susceptibility.[16]

4.2.4 Complement System Activation

The complement system plays a crucial role in opsonization and immune cell recruitment. However, unregulated activation of complement, especially through components like C3a and C5a, can exacerbate lung inflammation and damage. Local complement production, such as epithelial cell-derived C3, has been shown to play protective roles, but excessive activation remains harmful.[4]

Additionally, the lectin pathway of complement activation has been identified as a contributor to inflammatory lung damage, further demonstrating that tight regulation is necessary to avoid exacerbation of tissue injury.[5]

4.2.5 Immunological Biomarkers in sCAP

Evaluating both inflammatory and immunosuppressive biomarkers is crucial in determining the severity of sCAP and in guiding appropriate therapeutic interventions. Increased concentrations of inflammatory mediators such as interleukin-6 (IL-6), procalcitonin, and C-reactive protein (CRP) signal an active systemic inflammatory response and are linked to poorer clinical outcomes. In contrast, indicators of immune suppression, including reduced HLA-DR expression on monocytes and lymphopenia, reflect a state of immune exhaustion that predisposes patients to secondary infections and worsened prognosis.[1,2]

In addition to systemic markers, assessment of local immune function in the lungs provides valuable prognostic information. Research by Singh and colleagues found that reduced CD4+ T-cell levels in bronchoalveolar lavage fluid (BALF) were significantly associated with adverse clinical outcomes in sCAP patients. This suggests that impaired local adaptive immune responses may contribute to disease progression and mortality.[7] Consequently, the combination of systemic and localized immune biomarkers offers a more comprehensive strategy for identifying high-risk patients and tailoring immunomodulatory treatments.

4.2.6 Immune-Modulating Therapies

Therapeutic strategies aimed at targeting the host immune response are currently under investigation. Corticosteroids, IL-6 receptor blockers, and complement inhibitors are being studied for their potential to modulate excessive immune reactions. Additionally, intravenous immunoglobulin (IVIG) is gaining attention for its role in managing severe pneumonia. IVIG contains antibodies that enhance the immune response, normalize dysregulated immune activity, and neutralize toxins produced by pathogens like *Streptococcus pneumoniae*. This highlights the intricate interplay between pathogen factors and host immunity, which could be further explored for therapeutic targeting. Notably, pneumolysin from *Streptococcus pneumoniae* plays distinct roles in activating complement system and inducing cytotoxic effects, underscoring the complexity of the immune response in severe infections.[6]

While corticosteroids remain a cornerstone for dampening hyperinflammation, recent trials have explored IL-1 blockers (e.g., anakinra) and interferon gamma to reverse immunoparalysis. A phase II study showed that recombinant IFN-γ restored monocyte HLA-DR expression and improved bacterial clearance in septic patients with features of immune exhaustion, offering potential in selected sCAP cases.[17]

Another promising approach is anti-PD-1 therapy, typically used in oncology, repurposed to reinvigorate T-cell function in immunosuppressed ICU patients. Although early-phase data are limited, case reports suggest reversal of lymphocyte exhaustion and improved infection control with low-dose checkpoint blockade.[18]

Moreover, GM-CSF (granulocyte-macrophage colony-stimulating factor) has been evaluated as a means to boost alveolar macrophage function. In a pilot trial of patients with impaired monocyte HLA-DR expression,

GM-CSF administration led to partial immune restoration without excessive inflammation, warranting further trials in sCAP.[19]

4.3 Conclusion

Severe community-acquired pneumonia (sCAP) results from an imbalance between the host immune response and pathogen virulence. An excessive immune response can lead to lung damage, while immune suppression increases the risk of secondary infections. Both innate and adaptive immunity play crucial roles in defense but may also contribute to tissue injury if dysregulated. Biomarkers such as IL-6, CRP, and lymphocyte counts help assess disease severity and guide treatment decisions. Emerging therapies including corticosteroids, IL-6 blockers, complement inhibitors, and IVIG offer promising ways to restore immune balance and improve outcomes. A deeper understanding of immune mechanisms is essential to advancing the management of sCAP.

The discovery of microbiome–immune interactions, immune checkpoint upregulation, and new cellular players such as Mo-Macs and ILCs has deepened our understanding of sCAP. This growing knowledge base paves the way for targeted immunotherapies—ranging from IL-6 and complement blockade to immunostimulatory interventions like IFN-γ or GM-CSF that aim to rebalance host immunity. As personalized immunomodulation becomes more feasible, biomarker-guided therapy will be critical to optimizing outcomes in sCAP.

References

1. Huber-Lang M, Younes M, Huber B, El-Benna J, Bachem MG. The complement system in lung disease. *Cell Tissue Res.* 2018;374(3):567–591. Available from: https://www.ncbi.nlm.nih.gov/pmc/articles/PMC4189484/

2. Kulkarni HS, Elvington M, Perng YC, Liszewski MK, Byers DE, Farkouh C, et al. Lung epithelial cell-derived C3 protects against pneumonia-induced lung injury. *Sci Immunol.* 2019;4(40):eaap9547. Available from: doi:10.1126/sciimmunol.abp9547

3. Takahashi K, Iwaki D, Endo Y, Nakata M, Matsushita M. The influence of the lectin pathway of complement activation on the development of lung injury and inflammation. *Front Immunol.* 2020;11:585243. Available from: https://www.frontiersin.org/articles/10.3389/fimmu.2020.585243/full

4. Rubins JB, Charboneau D, Janoff EN. Distinct roles for pneumolysin's cytotoxic and complement activities during the pathogenesis of severe pneumococcal pneumonia. *Am J Respir Crit Care Med.* 1996;153(4 Pt 1):1339–1346. Available from: doi:10.1164/ajrccm.153.4.8616564

5. Ali YM, Lynch NJ, Haleem KS, Fujita T, Endo Y, Hansen S, et al. The lectin pathway of complement activation is a critical component of the innate immune response to pneumococcal infection. *PLoS Pathog.* 2012;8(7):e1002793. Available from: https://journals.plos.org/plospathogens/article?id=10.1371/journal.ppat.1002793

6. Hirst RA, Kadioglu A, O'Callaghan C, Andrew PW. The role of pneumolysin in pneumococcal pneumonia and meningitis. *Clin Exp Immunol.* 2004;138(2):195–201. Available from: https://academic.oup.com/cei/article/138/2/195/657372

7. Singh G, Martin Rumende C, Sharma SK, Rengganis I, Amin Z, Loho T, et al. Low CD4+ T-cell count in bronchoalveolar lavage fluid is associated with poor outcomes in severe community-acquired pneumonia. *J Crit Care.* 2021;63:192–197. Available from: doi:10.1080/07853890.2022.2095012

8. Westphalen K, Gusarova GA, Islam MN, Subramanian M, Cohen TS, Prince AS, et al. Sessile alveolar macrophages communicate with alveolar epithelium to modulate immunity. *Nature.* 2014;506(7489):503–506. Available from: https://www.nature.com/articles/nature12902

9. Guilliams M, De Kleer I, Henri S, Post S, Vanhoutte L, De Prijck S, et al. Alveolar macrophages develop from fetal monocytes that differentiate into long-lived cells

in the first week of life via GM-CSF. *Mucosal Immunol.* 2013;6(3):464. Available from: https://www.nature.com/articles/mi2012102

10. Whitsett JA, Alenghat T. Epithelial-macrophage interactions in lung homeostasis and disease. *Nat Immunol.* 2015;16(1):27–35. Available from: https://www.nature.com/articles/ni.3045

11. Demaria O, Cornen S, Daëron M, Morel Y, Medzhitov R, Vivier E. Natural killer cells in pneumonia: defenders and regulators. *Nature.* 2019;574(7776):45–56. Available from: https://www.nature.com/articles/s41586-019-1590-6

12. Hernández PP, Mahlakõiv T, Yang I, Schwierzeck V, Nguyen N, Guendel F, et al. Interleukin-22 and innate lymphoid cells in mucosal immunity. *Front Cell Infect Microbiol.* 2015;5:45. Available from: https://www.frontiersin.org/articles/10.3389/fcimb.2015.00045/full

13. Nakamura S, Davis KM, Weiser JN. Synergistic stimulation of type I interferons during influenza virus coinfection promotes Streptococcus pneumoniae colonization in mice. *Cell Host Microbe.* 2011;10(2):136–146. Available from: https://www.cell.com/cell-host-microbe/fulltext/S1931-3128(11)00217-7

14. Crotty S. Follicular helper CD4 T cells (Tfh). *Annu Rev Immunol.* 2011;29:621–663. Available from: doi:10.1146/annurev-immunol-031210-101400

15. Hotchkiss RS, Monneret G, Payen D. Sepsis-induced immunosuppression: from cellular dysfunctions to immunotherapy. *Nat Rev Immunol.* 2013;13(12):862–874. Available from: https://www.nature.com/articles/nri3552

16. Brudecki L, Ferguson DA, McCall CE, El Gazzar M. Myeloid-derived suppressor cells evolve during sepsis and can enhance or impair host immunity. *J Immunol.* 2012;189(9):4666–4675. Available from: https://www.jimmunol.org/content/189/9/4666.long

17. Meisel C, Schefold JC, Pschowski R, Baumann T, Hetzger K, Gregor J, et al. Granulocyte-macrophage colony-stimulating factor to reverse sepsis-associated immunosuppression: a double-blind, randomized, placebo-controlled multicenter trial. *Am J Respir Crit Care Med.* 2009;180(7):640–648. Available from: doi:10.1164/rccm.200903-0363OC

18. Weber GF, Chousterman BG, He S, Fenn AM, Nairz M, Anzai A, et al. Reversal of immunosuppression in sepsis by checkpoint inhibition: a pilot clinical trial. *N Engl J Med.* 2020;382(10):948–954.

19. Hotchkiss RS, Colston E, Yende S, Crouser ED, Martin GS, Albertson TE, et al. Immune checkpoint inhibition in sepsis: A phase 1b randomized study. *Nat Med.* 2019;25(11):1865–1873. Available from: https://www.nature.com/articles/s41591-019-0633-5

CHAPTER **5**

FAST HUGS BID

Addressing Severe Pneumonia with Prompt Intervention

5.1 Introduction

The management of patients with severe pneumonia in the intensive care unit (ICU) demands a multidimensional and evidence-based approach to reduce the risk of complications and improve clinical outcomes. Among various strategies developed to enhance the quality and consistency of critical care delivery, the FAST HUGS BID mnemonic has gained significant acceptance as a daily checklist to ensure that fundamental care elements are not overlooked. Originally introduced by Vincent and Hatton, this mnemonic encompasses crucial aspects of ICU care (Table 5.1).

5.2 Feeding

Nutritional support is a fundamental aspect of care in critically ill patients, particularly those with severe pneumonia, as it helps meet elevated metabolic demands and supports recovery. Early initiation of enteral nutrition,

 DOI:10.1201/9781003629504-5

TABLE 5.1 FAST HUGS BID Mnemonics

F	Feeding
A	Analgesia
S	Sedation
T	Thromboembolism prophylaxis
H	Head-of-bed elevation
U	Ulcer prophylaxis
G	Glycemic control
S	Spontaneous breathing trial
B	Bowel care
I	Indwelling catheter removal
D	De-escalation of antibiotics

ideally within 24 to 48 hours of ICU admission, has been associated with improved clinical outcomes, including reduced infection rates, shorter duration of mechanical ventilation, and decreased hospital length of stay.[1,2] Malnutrition remains a frequent issue and is linked with increased morbidity and mortality, emphasizing the need for timely nutritional interventions.[3]

The Nutrition Risk in Critically Ill (NUTRIC) score provides a structured assessment to identify patients most likely to benefit from aggressive nutritional support. It incorporates factors such as age, comorbidities, and organ dysfunction scores. A modified version excluding interleukin-6 (IL-6) has been introduced to facilitate practical bedside use.[4] According to ESPEN 2019 guidelines, early enteral nutrition is preferred in hemodynamically stable patients, with progressive increases in caloric and protein intake. A protein target of 1.3 g/kg/day is recommended to preserve muscle mass and improve outcomes, while the routine use of L-glutamine is not advised in patients with multiple organ failure or septic shock due to limited efficacy and potential adverse effects.[2]

A formulation containing meglumine sodium succinate has emerged as a promising adjunct in critically ill patients. It offers metabolic and antioxidant benefits and may serve as an alternative to L-glutamine, particularly in conditions involving oxidative stress and mitochondrial dysfunction. Preliminary findings support its role in modulating inflammation and improving cellular metabolism.[5]

Fluid resuscitation also plays a critical role in the early management of patients with septic shock due to severe pneumonia. Crystalloids, such as balanced salt solutions, remain the first-line choice due to availability and safety profile. Colloids, such as albumin 5% or 20–25%, may be considered in select cases—particularly in patients with hypoalbuminemia or persistent hemodynamic instability despite adequate crystalloid resuscitation. However, fluid therapy must be titrated carefully to avoid fluid overload and secondary complications like pulmonary edema.[6]

Evidence from the EPaNIC trial suggests that delaying parenteral nutrition during the early phase of critical illness may be associated with improved recovery, provided that enteral nutrition is initiated and progressively optimized.[7]

5.3 Analgesia

Effective pain management is crucial for critically ill patients, as unrelieved pain can result in complications such as agitation, delirium, immunosuppression, and prolonged mechanical ventilation. Additionally, it contributes to long-term psychological effects, including post-intensive care syndrome (PICS). Therefore, routine and reliable pain assessment is essential, especially in patients unable to communicate verbally, to ensure timely and appropriate analgesic interventions that enhance comfort and outcomes (Table 5.2).[8]

Behavioral Pain Scale (BPS): This scale is specifically designed for use in intubated and sedated patients in the ICU. It evaluates pain based on three behavioral indicators: facial expression, movements of the upper limbs, and

TABLE 5.2 Table of Behavioral Pain Scale (BPS)

Item	Description	Score
Facial expression	Relaxed	1
	Partially tightened (e.g., brow lowering)	2
	Fully tightened (e.g., eyelid closing)	3
	Grimacing	4
Upper limbs	No movement	1
	Partially bent	2
	Fully bent with finger flexion	3
	Permanently retracted	4
Compliance with ventilation	Tolerating movement	1
	Coughing with movement	2
	Fighting ventilator	3
	Unable to control ventilation	4

compliance with mechanical ventilation. Each domain is scored from 1 to 4, producing a total score ranging from 3 (no pain) to 12 (maximum pain). The BPS has demonstrated good inter-rater reliability and clinical utility for pain monitoring in non-communicative patients (Table 5.3).[9]

Critical-Care Pain Observation Tool (CPOT): CPOT is applicable to both intubated and extubated patients. It assesses pain based on four categories: facial expressions, body movements, muscle tension, and either compliance with the ventilator (for intubated patients) or vocalization (for extubated patients). Each item is rated from 0 to 2, yielding a total score between 0 and 8. CPOT is a widely validated instrument with strong psychometric properties, and it is recommended by critical care guidelines for routine pain assessment.[10]

Utilizing validated behavioral tools such as the BPS and CPOT enables clinicians to assess pain accurately,

TABLE 5.3 Table of Critical-Care Pain Observation Tool (CPOT)

Sub-scale	Description	Score
Facial expression	Relaxed, neutral	0
	Tense	1
	Grimacing	2
Body movements	Absence of movements	0
	Protection	1
	Restlessness	2
Muscle tension	Relaxed	0
	Tense, rigid	1
	Very tense or rigid	2
Compliance with ventilation	Tolerating ventilator or movement	0
	Coughing but tolerating	1
	Fighting ventilator	2
Vocalization (extubated patients)	Talking in normal tone or no sound	0
	Sighing, moaning	1
	Crying out, sobbing	2

even in sedated and mechanically ventilated patients, ensuring that analgesia is both adequate and individualized to improve clinical outcomes.[8–10]

5.4 Sedation

Sedation is a critical component in the management of ICU patients, especially those requiring mechanical ventilation. The primary goals of sedation are to ensure patient comfort, reduce anxiety, facilitate synchronization with the ventilator, and prevent accidental removal of life-support equipment. However, inappropriate sedation—either under-sedation or over-sedation can result in adverse outcomes, including prolonged mechanical ventilation, increased ICU length of stay, and a higher incidence of ICU-related delirium. Appropriate sedation practices are

TABLE 5.4   Richmond Agitation–Sedation Scale (RASS)

Score	Term	Description
4	Combative	Overtly combative, violent, immediate danger to staff
3	Very agitated	Pulls or removes tubes or catheters; aggressive
2	Agitated	Frequent non-purposeful movement, fights ventilator
1	Restless	Anxious but movements not aggressive or vigorous
0	Alert and calm	
	Drowsy	Sustained awakening to voice (≥10 sec)
−2	Light sedation	Briefly awakens with eye contact to voice (<10 sec)
−3	Moderate sedation	Movement or eye opening to voice but no eye contact
−4	Deep sedation	No response to voice but movement or eye opening to physical stimulation
−5	Cannot be aroused	No response to voice or physical

integral to improving patient outcomes and minimizing complications in critically ill patients (Table 5.4).[8–11]

To ensure optimal sedation, validated tools such as the Richmond Agitation–Sedation Scale (RASS) are widely recommended. RASS is a 10-point scale, ranging from +4 (combative) to −5 (unarousable). It is used to assess both agitation and sedation levels in critically ill patients. The ideal sedation target for most ICU patients is typically a RASS score between −2 (light sedation) and 0 (alert and calm). Regular assessment using RASS enables clinicians to titrate sedative agents more accurately, avoiding unnecessarily deep sedation that has been associated with longer mechanical ventilation duration and poor neurological outcomes.[12–13]

In summary, careful and regular assessment of sedation using tools like RASS, combined with evidence-based strategies such as daily sedation interruption and early mobilization, can enhance patient safety, reduce ICU length of stay, and facilitate early recovery.[8-13]

5.5 Thromboprophylaxis

Critically ill patients in the ICU are at an increased risk of venous thromboembolism (VTE), including deep vein thrombosis (DVT) and pulmonary embolism (PE), due to factors such as immobility, systemic inflammation, mechanical ventilation, and central venous catheters. VTE significantly contributes to morbidity, mortality, and prolonged hospital stays, necessitating effective preventive measures.[14]

Pharmacologic thromboprophylaxis, primarily using low molecular weight heparin (LMWH) or unfractionated heparin (UFH), is the mainstay of VTE prevention in critically ill patients. These agents have been shown to reduce the occurrence of thrombotic events. For patients with a high risk of bleeding, mechanical thromboprophylaxis, such as intermittent pneumatic compression (IPC) or graduated compression stockings (GCS), offers a safe alternative to enhance venous return and prevent stasis.[15]

For patients transitioning out of critical illness who remain at high risk for thromboembolic events, the use of direct oral anticoagulants (DOACs) like apixaban, rivaroxaban, and dabigatran offers an effective strategy for extended thromboprophylaxis. These agents are advantageous due to their ease of administration, predictable pharmacokinetics, and lack of routine monitoring. Extended use of DOACs has been shown to reduce the risk of recurrent VTE and prevent chronic complications, such as chronic thromboembolic pulmonary hypertension (CTEPH) in post-PE patients. However, the decision to use DOACs for extended thromboprophylaxis should be individualized, with careful consideration

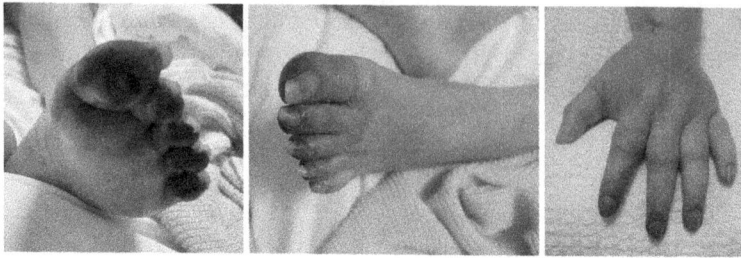

FIGURE 5.1 Clinical manifestation of limb ischemia due to massive thrombosis in a patient with severe community-acquired pneumonia.

of the patient's bleeding risk and clinical condition.[16,17] Severe thrombotic events in critically ill patients, if not promptly recognized and managed, can result in devastating complications such as peripheral ischemia and tissue necrosis. Figure 5.1 illustrates a striking example of acral ischemia in a patient with severe community-acquired pneumonia, underscoring the urgency of early and adequate thromboprophylaxis.

In conclusion, a combined approach of pharmacologic and mechanical thromboprophylaxis during the acute phase, followed by tailored extended prophylaxis with DOACs, is essential to minimize thromboembolic complications and improve outcomes for critically ill patients.

5.6 Head-of-Bed Elevation

Maintaining the head of the bed at an elevation of 30 to 45 degrees is a well-established and evidence-based intervention aimed at preventing aspiration and ventilator-associated pneumonia (VAP), particularly in critically ill patients undergoing mechanical ventilation. The semi-recumbent position improves respiratory mechanics, facilitates diaphragmatic movement, reduces gastroesophageal reflux, and decreases the risk of aspiration of gastric contents into the lower airways. Elevating the head of the bed is not only critical for pulmonary protection but also enhances enteral feeding tolerance and reduces the incidence of gastrointestinal complications such as regurgitation and aspiration. This reinforces the multidisciplinary relevance of this simple intervention, spanning both respiratory and nutritional domains of intensive care (Figure 5.2).[6]

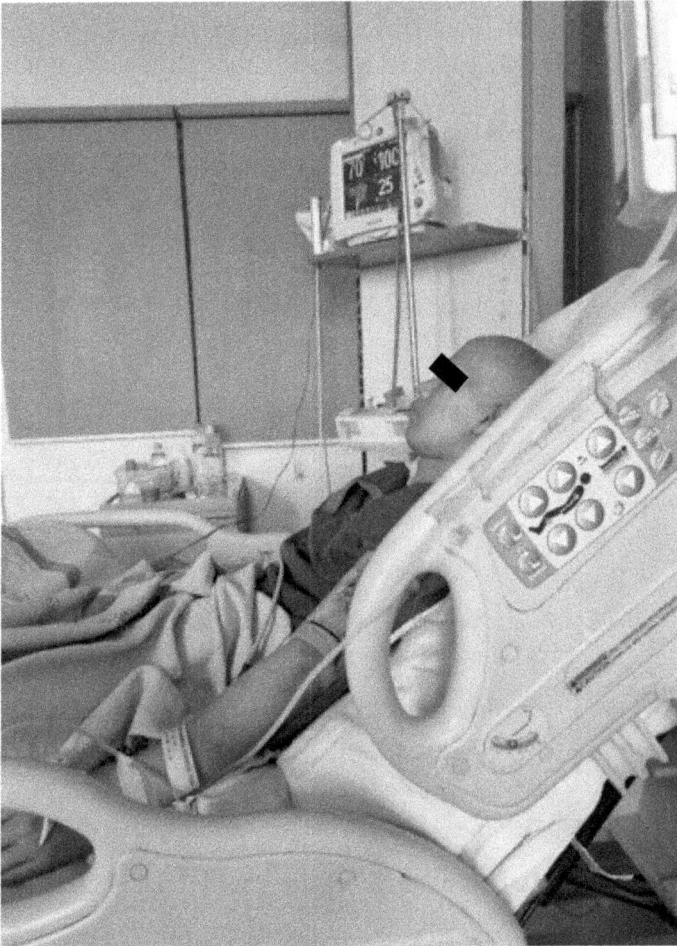

FIGURE 5.2 Patient on head-of-bed elevation.

5.7 Ulcer Prophylaxis

Stress ulcer prophylaxis in critically ill patients is intended to prevent gastrointestinal (GI) bleeding resulting from stress-related mucosal damage, particularly in those with impaired mucosal perfusion or increased acid production. The *BMJ* clinical practice guideline recommends a more judicious, risk-based approach to prophylaxis.[18]

Routine pharmacologic prophylaxis is not indicated for all ICU patients, especially those who are not enterally fed and lack significant bleeding risk factors. Instead, prophylaxis should be reserved for patients at high risk of clinically significant GI bleeding, including:

- Mechanical ventilation for >48 hours
- Coagulopathy (platelet count <50,000/mm³, INR >1.5, or aPTT >2× normal)
- History of peptic ulcer or GI bleeding within the past year
- Severe burns (>35% total body surface area)
- Traumatic brain or spinal cord injury
- Multiple trauma
- Hypoperfusion states (e.g., shock, sepsis, organ failure)[6]

In patients meeting these criteria, the following pharmacological agents are commonly used:

a. Proton Pump Inhibitors (PPIs)
- Pantoprazole 40 mg IV once daily
- Esomeprazole 40 mg IV once daily
- Omeprazole 20–40 mg orally or IV once daily

b. Histamine-2 Receptor Antagonists (H2RAs)
- Ranitidine 50 mg IV every 8 hours (note: limited use due to global shortages and regulatory restrictions)
- Famotidine 20 mg IV every 12 hours

TABLE 5.5   Evidence Profile Comparing Proton Pump Inhibitors (PPIs) and Histamine-2 Receptor Antagonists (H2RAs)

Outcome	Better Option	Effect	Evidence Quality
Important bleeding (1–2% risk)	No difference	No important difference	Low
Important bleeding (2–4% risk)	PPI	13 fewer cases per 1000 people	Low
Important bleeding (4–8% risk)	PPI	37 fewer cases per 1000 people	Moderate
Important bleeding (8–10% risk)	PPI	57 fewer cases per 1000 people	Moderate
Mortality	No difference	Similar death rates	Very low
Pneumonia	No difference	Similar infection rates	Low
Clostridium difficile infection	No difference	Similar rates	Low
Length of stay in intensive care	No difference	Almost identical (7.4 vs 7.3 days)	High

PPIs are generally preferred in high-risk patients due to superior acid suppression, although concerns remain regarding associations with ventilator-associated pneumonia (VAP) and *Clostridioides difficile* infection.[17] When feasible, early enteral nutrition is recommended as a non-pharmacologic protective factor and may reduce the need for pharmacologic prophylaxis (Table 5.5).[1,2,17]

5.8 Glycemic Control

Glycemic control represents a critical aspect of metabolic management in critically ill patients. Stress-induced hyperglycemia is a common occurrence in the ICU, even among non-diabetic individuals, due to the counter-regulatory hormonal response involving cortisol, glucagon, and catecholamines. These hormones promote insulin resistance and increased hepatic glucose output, leading to elevated blood glucose levels.[19]

Optimal glycemic control in the ICU should aim to maintain blood glucose levels within a moderate target range of 140–180 mg/dL, rather than pursuing tight glycemic control (80–110 mg/dL), which has been associated with an increased risk of hypoglycemia and related adverse outcomes. This recommendation is in alignment with contemporary critical care guidelines, emphasizing a balance between avoiding both hyperglycemia and hypoglycemia.[19]

In practice, glycemic control requires regular blood glucose monitoring typically every 4 to 6 hours and the use of insulin protocols that may include intravenous or subcutaneous insulin, tailored to individual patient needs. Nutritional interventions, including the timing and composition of enteral or parenteral nutrition, must be carefully coordinated with insulin therapy to prevent glycemic fluctuations. Effective glycemic control is essential not only for metabolic stability but also for reducing infection risk, improving wound healing, and optimizing overall outcomes in critically ill patients.[19]

5.9 Spontaneous Breathing Trial

The Spontaneous Breathing Trial (SBT) is an essential step in the process of weaning patients from mechanical ventilation. It evaluates the patient's ability to breathe independently without ventilatory support, typically conducted with low levels of Continuous Positive Airway Pressure (CPAP) or a T-piece for 30–120 minutes. A successful SBT is defined by the absence of respiratory distress signs such as tachypnea, oxygen desaturation, or hypercapnia. The trial should be performed only in hemodynamically stable patients without contraindications like severe hypoxemia, acidosis, or active infections.[20,21]

Besides common causes like respiratory muscle fatigue and malnutrition, diaphragmatic dysfunction plays a significant role in SBT failure. Diaphragmatic paralysis diminishes ventilatory capacity, even in patients clinically ready for extubation, and may result from phrenic nerve injury, critical illness neuromyopathy, or after thoracic and cervical surgeries.[22,23]

Ultrasonography offers a practical, non-invasive bedside approach to assess diaphragm function. M-mode ultrasound measures diaphragmatic excursion and thickening fraction, indicators of diaphragm contractility. An excursion less than 10 mm or a thickening fraction below 20–30% suggests dysfunction and predicts weaning failure. Using diaphragm ultrasound during SBT provides valuable diagnostic information to identify high-risk patients and guide treatment strategies.[24,25]

5.10 Bowel Care

Bowel care is essential in ICU patients as gastrointestinal issues like constipation and ileus frequently occur due to immobility, sedatives, opioids, and critical illness itself. These complications can worsen feeding intolerance and increase the risk of further morbidity.[26,27]

The gut–lung axis plays a significant role in critical illness. Disruption of the intestinal barrier allows bacteria and toxins to translocate into the bloodstream and lungs, triggering inflammation and worsening lung injury, contributing to sepsis and ARDS.[28,29]

Gut and lung microbiomes are crucial for immune regulation. Dysbiosis is common in ICU patients and may impair immune defenses, increasing susceptibility to lung infections. Supporting a balanced microbiome may reduce inflammation and improve respiratory outcomes.[30,31]

Probiotics such as *Lactobacillus reuteri* have shown potential to restore gut balance by reducing harmful bacteria, enhancing barrier function, and modulating immunity, which may benefit critically ill patients.[32,33]

Managing the gut microbiome with probiotics, adequate nutrition, and cautious antibiotic use can help prevent complications by limiting microbial translocation and supporting gut and lung health. Bowel care is a key part of ICU management, not only to prevent gastrointestinal complications but also to support respiratory recovery and reduce systemic inflammation.[34,35]

5.11 Indwelling Catheter Removal

The prolonged use of indwelling medical devices, including urinary catheters and central venous catheters (CVCs), is a well-established risk factor for healthcare-associated infections. Catheter-associated urinary tract infections (CAUTIs) and central line-associated bloodstream infections (CLABSIs) contribute substantially to patient morbidity, extended hospitalization, and increased healthcare costs. These infections often result from prolonged catheterization or lapses in aseptic technique during insertion or maintenance procedures (Figure 5.3).[36,37]

One preventive strategy for CAUTIs includes the intravesical administration of hyaluronic acid and chondroitin sulfate. These agents help restore the bladder's glycosaminoglycan (GAG) layer and reduce urothelial inflammation, and may limit bacterial adherence. Several studies have demonstrated their effectiveness in patients with recurrent or complicated urinary tract infections.[38,39]

Clinically, it is essential to reassess the necessity of catheters regularly. Prompt removal of unnecessary catheters, adherence to aseptic insertion and maintenance protocols, and close monitoring for signs of infection are vital steps

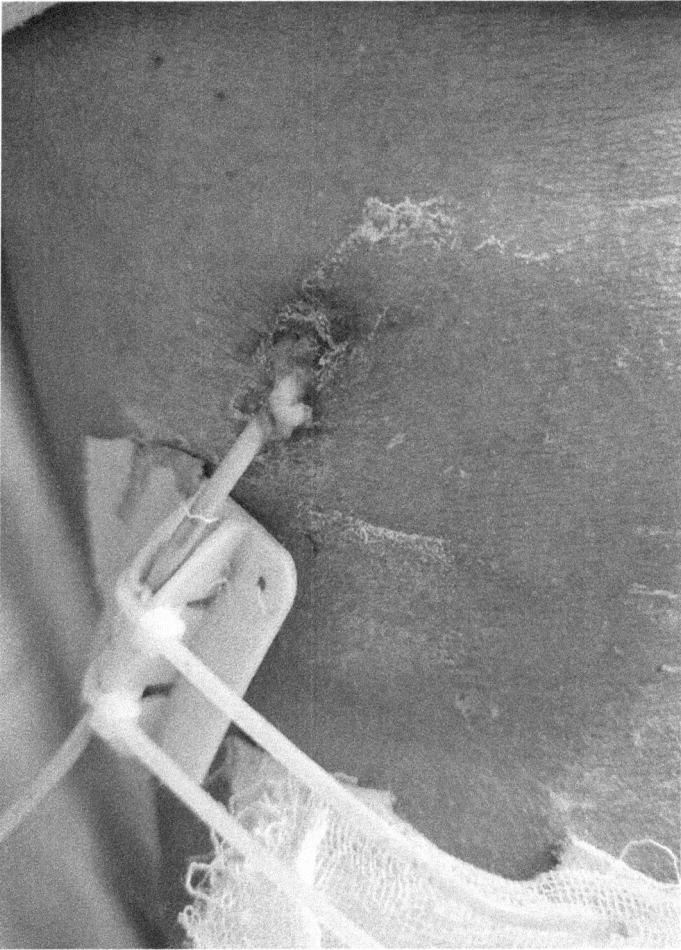

FIGURE 5.3 Patient with central line-associated bloodstream infections (CLABSIs).

in preventing catheter-associated complications. Where appropriate, intravesical therapy with hyaluronic acid and chondroitin sulfate may provide additional benefits as part of a comprehensive infection prevention strategy.[40]

5.12 De-escalation of Antibiotics

Antibiotic de-escalation refers to the practice of reducing the spectrum or discontinuing antimicrobial therapy based on microbiological findings, clinical improvement, or the absence of a confirmed infection. This strategy helps mitigate antimicrobial resistance, reduce adverse drug effects, and lower healthcare costs without compromising patient safety or treatment efficacy.[41]

Critically ill patients, particularly those with severe pneumonia, often receive broad-spectrum antibiotics empirically due to the urgency and potential severity of infection. However, once clinical stability is achieved and microbiology results become available typically within 48–72 hours therapy should be reassessed and narrowed to target specific pathogens, or discontinued if infection is not confirmed. Evidence supports that de-escalation is both safe and beneficial, with studies showing reduced ICU stay, lower healthcare-associated complications, and decreased incidence of *Clostridioides difficile* infection.[42,43]

5.13 Conclusion

The FAST HUGS BID mnemonic serves as a critical framework for ensuring comprehensive and standardized care in patients with severe pneumonia in the ICU. By systematically addressing key components such as nutrition, pain and sedation management, thromboprophylaxis, positioning, ulcer and glycemic control, weaning readiness, bowel function, catheter care, and antibiotic stewardship, this checklist reinforces evidence-based best practices. Each element not only targets specific risks but also contributes to holistic patient stabilization and recovery. Implementing FAST HUGS BID on a daily basis helps minimize complications, optimize resource use, and improve clinical outcomes, making it an indispensable tool in modern critical care management for severe pneumonia.

References

1. McClave SA, Taylor BE, Martindale RG, Warren MM, Johnson DR, Braunschweig C, et al. Guidelines for the provision and assessment of nutrition support therapy in the adult critically ill patient: Society of Critical Care Medicine (SCCM) and American Society for Parenteral and Enteral Nutrition (ASPEN). *JPEN J Parenter Enteral Nutr.* 2016;40(2):159–211. doi:10.1177/0148607115621863
2. Singer P, Blaser AR, Berger MM, Alhazzani W, Calder PC, Casaer MP, et al. ESPEN guideline on clinical nutrition in the intensive care unit. *Clin Nutr.* 2019;38(1):48–79. doi:10.1016/j.clnu.2018.08.037
3. Correia MI, Waitzberg DL. The impact of malnutrition on morbidity, mortality, length of hospital stay and costs evaluated through a multivariate model analysis. *Clin Nutr.* 2003;22(3):235–239. doi:10.1016/S0261-5614(02)00215-7
4. Rahman A, Hasan RM, Agarwala R, Martin C, Day AG, Heyland DK. Identifying critically ill patients who will benefit most from nutritional therapy: Further validation of the "modified NUTRIC" nutritional risk assessment tool. *Clin Nutr.* 2016;35(1):158–162. doi:10.1016/j.clnu.2015.01.015
5. Kagan VE, Tyurin VA, Jiang J, Tyurina YY, Mohammadyani D, Angeli JP, et al. Antioxidant defense and repair mechanisms in response to the ferroptosis-like cell death in critical illness: Potential role of succinate-based agents. *Biochim Biophys Acta Mol Basis Dis.* 2020;1866(10):165765. doi:10.1016/j.bbadis.2020.165765
6. Rhodes A, Evans LE, Alhazzani W, Levy MM, Antonelli M, Ferrer R, et al. Surviving sepsis campaign: International guidelines for management of sepsis and septic shock: 2016. *Intensive Care Med.* 2017;43(3):304–377. doi:10.1007/s00134-017-4683-6
7. Casaer MP, Mesotten D, Hermans G, Wouters PJ, Schetz M, Meyfroidt G, et al. Early versus late parenteral nutrition in critically ill adults. *N Engl J Med.* 2011;365(6):506–517. doi:10.1056/NEJMoa1102662

8. Barr J, Fraser GL, Puntillo K, Ely EW, Gélinas C, Dasta JF, et al. Clinical practice guidelines for the management of pain, agitation, and delirium in adult patients in the intensive care unit. *Crit Care Med.* 2013;41(1):263–306. doi:10.1097/CCM.0b013e3182783b72

9. Payen JF, Bru O, Bosson JL, Lagrasta A, Novel E, Deschaux I, et al. Assessing pain in critically ill sedated patients by using a Behavioral Pain Scale. *Crit Care Med.* 2001;29(12):2258–2263. doi:10.1097/00003246-200112000-00004

10. Gélinas C, Fillion L, Puntillo KA, Viens C, Fortier M. Validation of the critical-care pain observation tool in adult patients. *Am J Crit Care.* 2006;15(4):420–427. doi:10.4037/ajcc2006.15.4.420

11. Reade MC, Finfer S. Sedation and delirium in the intensive care unit. *N Engl J Med.* 2014;370(5):444–454. doi:10.1056/NEJMra1208705

12. Sessler CN, Gosnell MS, Grap MJ, Brophy GM, O'Neal PV, Keane KA, et al. The Richmond Agitation–Sedation Scale: validity and reliability in adult intensive care unit patients. *Am J Respir Crit Care Med.* 2002;166(10):1338–1344. doi:10.1164/rccm.2107138

13. Kress JP, Pohlman AS, O'Connor MF, Hall JB. Daily interruption of sedative infusions in critically ill patients undergoing mechanical ventilation. *N Engl J Med.* 2000;342(20):1471–1477. doi:10.1056/NEJM200005183422002

14. Cook DJ, Meade MO, Guyatt GH, Walter SD, Heels-Ansdell D, Warkentin TE, et al. Dalteparin versus unfractionated heparin in critically ill patients. *N Engl J Med.* 2011;364(14):1305–1314. doi:10.1056/NEJMoa1014475

15. Geerts WH, Bergqvist D, Pineo GF, Heit JA, Samama CM, Lassen MR, et al. Prevention of venous thromboembolism: American College of Chest Physicians Evidence-Based Clinical Practice Guidelines (8th Edition). *Chest.* 2008;133(6 Suppl):381S–453S. doi:10.1378/chest.08-0656

16. Spyropoulos AC, Lipardi C, Xu J, Peluso C, Spiro TE, De Sanctis Y, et al. Improved benefit-risk profile of extended-duration rivaroxaban thromboprophylaxis in acutely ill medical patients: A post hoc analysis of the MAGELLAN study. *Thromb Haemost.* 2019;119(6):1031–1040. doi:10.1055/s-0039-1688444

17. Drakulovic MB, Torres A, Bauer TT, Nicolas JM, Nogué S, Ferrer M. Supine body position as a risk factor for nosocomial pneumonia in mechanically ventilated patients: A randomized trial. *Lancet*. 1999;354(9193):1851–1858. doi:10.1016/S0140-6736(98)12251-1

18. Ye Z, Reintam Blaser A, Lytvyn L, Wang Y, Guyatt GH, Mikita JS, et al. Gastrointestinal bleeding prophylaxis for critically ill patients: a clinical practice guideline. *BMJ*. 2020;368:l6722. doi:10.1136/bmj.l6722

19. American Diabetes Association. 16. Diabetes care in the hospital: Standards of Medical Care in Diabetes—2024. *Diabetes Care*. 2024;47(Suppl 1):S295–S302. doi:10.2337/dc24-S016

20. MacIntyre NR, Cook DJ, Ely EW Jr, Epstein SK, Fink JB, Heffner JE, et al. Evidence-based guidelines for weaning and discontinuing ventilatory support: A collective task force facilitated by the American College of Chest Physicians; the American Association for Respiratory Care; and the American College of Critical Care Medicine. *Chest*. 2001;120(6 Suppl):375S–395S. doi:10.1378/chest.120.6_suppl.375s

21. Ely EW, Baker AM, Dunagan DP, Burke HL, Smith AC, Kelly PT, et al. Effect on the duration of mechanical ventilation of identifying patients capable of breathing spontaneously. *N Engl J Med*. 1996;335(25):1864–1869. doi:10.1056/NEJM199612193352502

22. Goligher EC, Laghi F, Detsky ME, Pinto R, Gopalakrishnan R, Fan E, et al. Measuring diaphragm thickness with ultrasound in mechanically ventilated patients: Feasibility, reproducibility and validity. *Intensive Care Med*. 2015;41(4):642–649.

23. Laghi F, Tobin MJ. Disorders of the respiratory muscles. *Am J Respir Crit Care Med*. 2003;168(1):10–48. doi:10.1164/rccm.2206008

24. Kim WY, Suh HJ, Hong SB, Oh Y, Lim CM. Diaphragm dysfunction assessed by ultrasonography: Influence on weaning from mechanical ventilation. *Crit Care Med*. 2011;39(12):2627–2630. doi:10.1097/CCM.0b013e3182266408

25. Supinski GS, Callahan LA. Diaphragm weakness in mechanically ventilated critically ill patients. *Crit Care*. 2013;17(3):R120. doi:10.1186/cc12770

26. Reintam Blaser A, Malbrain ML, Starkopf J, et al. Gastrointestinal function in intensive care patients: Terminology, definitions and management. Recommendations of the ESICM Working Group on Abdominal Problems. *Intensive Care Med.* 2012;38(3): 384–394.

27. Lewis SR, Pritchard MW, Thomas CM, et al. Early enteral nutrition within 24 hours of adult intensive care unit admission: A systematic review and meta-analysis. *J Crit Care.* 2020;60:119–127. doi:10.1016/j.jcrc.2020.05.002

28. Dickson RP. The microbiome and critical illness. *Lancet Respir Med.* 2016;4(1):59–72.

29. Enaud R, Prevel R, Ciarlo E, et al. The gut–lung axis in health and respiratory diseases: a place for inter-organ and inter-kingdom crosstalks. *Front Cell Infect Microbiol.* 2020;10:19. doi:10.3389/fcimb.2020.00009

30. Wypych TP, Marsland BJ, Levy BD. The lung microbiome and its role in respiratory health and disease. *Annu Rev Physiol.* 2019;81:481–504.

31. Mielcarek M, Vitkauskiene A, Bitautiene J, et al. Role of gut microbiota in lung health and disease. *Curr Allergy Asthma Rep.* 2021;21(3):11.

32. Wischmeyer PE. Probiotics and critical illness: from synbiotics to fecal microbiota transplantation. *Curr Opin Crit Care.* 2018;24(2):83–88. doi:10.1097/MCC. 0000000000000472

33. Szajewska H, Skórka A. Meta-analysis: *Lactobacillus reuteri* DSM 17938 in the prevention of antibiotic-associated diarrhoea in children. *Aliment Pharmacol Ther.* 2015;42(8):964–972. doi:10.1111/apt.13321

34. Geng Z, Zhang X, Jin X, et al. Gut microbiota influence in critical illness: new therapeutic options. *J Crit Care.* 2021;65:40–48. doi:10.1016/j.jcrc.2021.02.010

35. Shimizu K, Ogura H, Goto M, et al. Altered gut flora and environment in patients with severe systemic inflammatory response syndrome. *JPEN J Parenter Enteral Nutr.* 2011;35(5):630–636.

36. Centers for Disease Control and Prevention. Catheter-associated Urinary Tract Infection (CAUTI) Basics. https://www.cdc.gov/uti/about/cauti-basics.html

37. Centers for Disease Control and Prevention. Central Line-associated Bloodstream Infection (CLABSI) Basics. https://www.cdc.gov/clabsi/about/index.html
38. Damiano R, et al. Intravesical hyaluronic acid and chondroitin sulfate for recurrent urinary tract infections: a systematic review. *Int Urogynecol J.* 2014;25(5):531–538.
39. De Vita D, Giordano S. Efficacy of intravesical hyaluronic acid and chondroitin sulfate in recurrent urinary tract infections: A meta-analysis. *Pain Ther.* 2023;12(1):45–56.
40. Riedl CR, et al. Intravesical administration of combined hyaluronic acid and chondroitin sulfate reduces the risk of recurrent urinary tract infections. *BMJ Open.* 2016;6(3):e009669.
41. Weiss E, Zahar JR, Lesprit P, et al. Elaboration of a consensual definition of de-escalation allowing a ranking of β-lactams. *Clin Microbiol Infect.* 2015;21(7):649.e1.
42. Garnacho-Montero J, Gutiérrez-Pizarraya A, Escoresca-Ortega A, Corcia-Palomo Y, Fernández-Delgado E, Herrera-Melero I. De-escalation of empirical therapy is associated with lower mortality in patients with severe sepsis and septic shock. *Intensive Care Med.* 2014;40(1):32–40.
43. Tabah A, Cotta MO, Garnacho-Montero J, et al. A systematic review of the definitions, determinants, and clinical outcomes of antimicrobial de-escalation in the intensive care unit. *Clin Infect Dis.* 2020;70(6):1173–1181.

CHAPTER **6**

The Clinical Impact of Early Bronchoscopy and Early Tracheostomy in Severe Community-Acquired Pneumonia

6.1 Introduction

Severe community-acquired pneumonia (sCAP) is a major global cause of acute respiratory failure and sepsis, often requiring intensive care unit (ICU) admission and mechanical ventilation. Mortality rates in sCAP can exceed 30%, particularly in patients with delayed antibiotic administration, inappropriate initial therapy, or unresolved airway obstruction.[1,2] The management of sCAP is further complicated by airway mucus hypersecretion, frequent polymicrobial etiology, and evolving antimicrobial resistance patterns. In this context, early procedural interventions, such as bronchoscopy and tracheostomy, have gained increasing attention as adjunctive measures to optimize respiratory support and improve patient-centered outcomes.[3]

 DOI:10.1201/9781003629504-6

Early bronchoscopy can assist not only in relieving airway obstruction but also in identifying causative pathogens more accurately, especially in settings where conventional sputum cultures are limited by contamination or insufficient yield. Likewise, early tracheostomy may mitigate the risk of ventilator-associated pneumonia (VAP), reduce sedation exposure, and facilitate communication and mobilization, thereby accelerating recovery.[4]

6.2 Early Bronchoscopy in Severe Community-Acquired Pneumonia

Bronchoscopy plays a crucial role in the diagnostic and therapeutic management of severe pneumonia. In sCAP patients requiring mechanical ventilation, bronchoscopic evaluation within 72 hours of intubation, termed early bronchoscopy, offers several advantages. Mechanistically, bronchoscopy allows for direct visualization and mechanical clearance of secretions, fibrinous debris, and mucus plugs that may occlude segmental or subsegmental airways. This improves ventilation–perfusion matching and reduces the risk of atelectasis and secondary bacterial overgrowth.[5]

Therapeutically, bronchoalveolar lavage (BAL) obtained during early bronchoscopy improves the accuracy of microbiological diagnosis by reducing contamination from upper respiratory flora and enabling detection of atypical pathogens or mixed infections. Studies using retrospective cohorts and ICU databases (e.g., MIMIC-IV) have shown that early bronchoscopy is associated with shorter durations of mechanical ventilation, earlier de-escalation of antibiotics, and reduced ICU stays.[6,7]

An analysis of the MIMIC-IV database of patients with severe pneumonia in intensive care units defined early bronchoscopy as within 3 days of ICU admission and found no significant difference in 28-day mortality, although bronchoscopy may facilitate pathogen identification and airway clearance.[8] Such findings suggest that early bronchoscopy can be particularly valuable in settings with high burden of multidrug-resistant organisms or pandemic-related diagnostic delays (Figures 6.1 and 6.2).

However, early bronchoscopy is not without risks. In patients with hemodynamic instability, severe hypoxemia, or high ventilator dependency, procedural sedation and bronchoscope-induced airway resistance may precipitate transient desaturation or cardiac compromise. Therefore, careful patient selection and close monitoring are mandatory. Furthermore, the diagnostic yield of

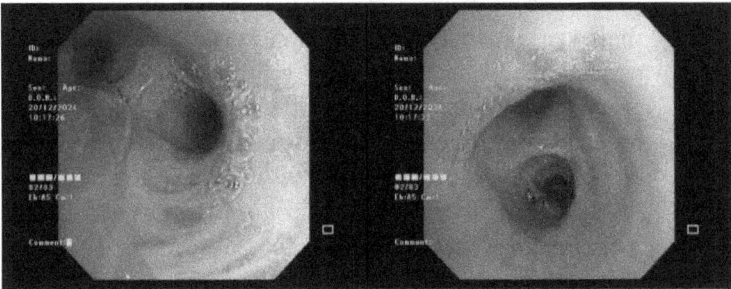

FIGURE 6.1 A bronchoscopic view showing extensive mucus obstruction in a mechanically ventilated sCAP patient.

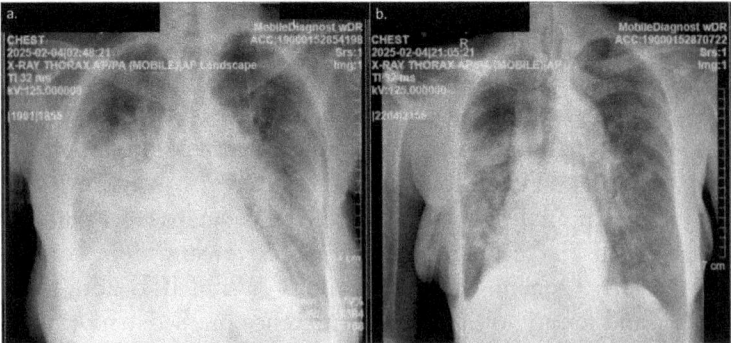

FIGURE 6.2 Serial chest X-rays pre- and post-bronchoscopy, demonstrating radiologic improvement following airway clearance.

BAL may be limited in patients who have received broad-spectrum antibiotics prior to the procedure.[9]

A prospective observational study in Germany emphasized that timing, operator expertise, and infection control protocols significantly influence the safety and effectiveness of bronchoscopy in the ICU.[10] Thus, integration of early bronchoscopy into sCAP management algorithms should be guided by individualized assessment, balancing potential diagnostic and therapeutic benefits with procedural risks. A detailed visualization related to this section is provided in the supplementary video (https://drive.google.com/file/d/1pAkUPxsz6iYzHd_SCskYeTc7Sd4S9Jvr/view?usp=sharing).

6.3 Early Tracheostomy in Severe Community-Acquired Pneumonia

Tracheostomy is frequently indicated in critically ill patients requiring prolonged mechanical ventilation. Conventionally, this procedure is performed after 10 to 14 days of endotracheal intubation; however, increasing evidence supports the benefits of early tracheostomy, typically defined as placement within the first 7 days of mechanical ventilation. In the context of sCAP, early tracheostomy may be particularly advantageous due to its association with improved pulmonary hygiene, earlier weaning from mechanical ventilation, reduced incidence of VAP, and enhanced patient comfort.[11]

Mechanistically, early tracheostomy decreases upper airway resistance, facilitates secretion clearance, and allows for more effective implementation of spontaneous breathing trials. The use of tracheostomy has been associated with reduced sedation requirements, lower rates of laryngeal injury, and earlier initiation of speech and physical rehabilitation in ICU patients.[12] In sCAP, where airway inflammation and mucus burden are often prominent, these advantages may translate to meaningful reductions in ICU length of stay and improved outcomes.

A multicenter cohort study reported that patients with sCAP who underwent early tracheostomy had significantly shorter durations of mechanical ventilation and ICU admission compared to those receiving late tracheostomy.[13] Furthermore, early tracheostomy was associated with fewer episodes of VAP, likely due to decreased microaspiration and improved oropharyngeal hygiene.[14]

Despite these benefits, the decision to perform early tracheostomy must be individualized. Predicting the need for prolonged ventilation remains a clinical challenge. Scores such as APACHE II, SOFA, or the Integrative Weaning Index (IWI) may assist in prognostication, but none offer absolute predictive accuracy.[15] Thus, patient factors such as comorbidities, baseline functional status, and response to initial therapy must be taken into account.

Two primary techniques for tracheostomy—percutaneous dilatational tracheostomy (PDT) and open surgical tracheostomy—are both used in the ICU setting. Meta-analyses show comparable complication rates, although PDT is often favored for bedside use due to reduced need for transport and shorter procedural time.[16] However, in sCAP patients with distorted neck anatomy, coagulopathy, or high oxygen demand, surgical tracheostomy may still be preferred.[17] Operator experience and institutional protocols should guide procedural choice (Figure 6.3).

6.4 Integrating Early Bronchoscopy and Early Tracheostomy

While early bronchoscopy and tracheostomy have independently demonstrated clinical benefit in sCAP, their combined application may offer additive or even synergistic effects—especially in patients with high secretion burden, prolonged ventilator dependency, or difficult-to-treat pathogens.[18]

Early bronchoscopy contributes to diagnostic accuracy and airway hygiene in the acute phase, while early

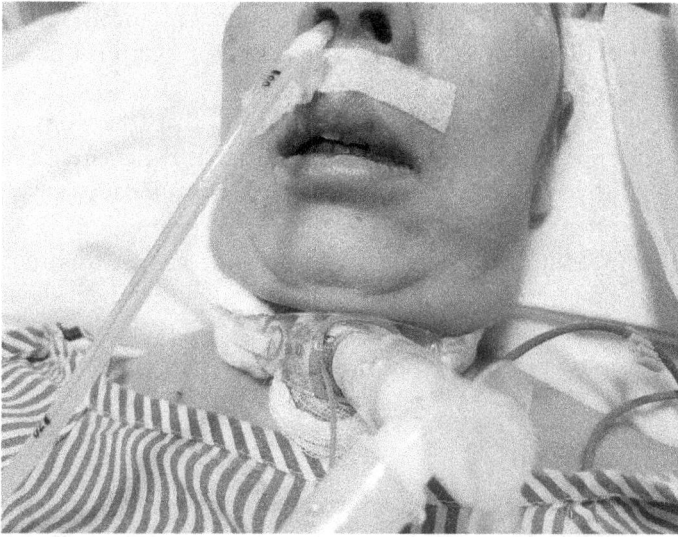

FIGURE 6.3 A tracheostomy tube *in situ* for prolonged ventilation in a patient with sCAP.

tracheostomy supports ongoing respiratory care and facilitates earlier rehabilitation. When performed in close succession within the first week of mechanical ventilation, these procedures may optimize respiratory mechanics, improve oxygenation, and reduce systemic inflammation secondary to impaired airway clearance or inappropriate antimicrobial therapy.[19] For instance, bronchoscopy-guided pathogen identification allows tailored antimicrobial de-escalation, while tracheostomy allows for safer implementation of spontaneous breathing trials and enhances ventilator weaning efforts.[20]

Emerging observational data from Asian ICU cohorts have shown that sCAP patients receiving both interventions early had shorter total ventilator days and ICU stays compared to those receiving only one or neither.[21] Additionally, these patients demonstrated lower rates of secondary nosocomial infections, likely due to improved secretion control and reduced sedation exposure.[22] However, such integrated strategies remain underutilized, likely due to variation in institutional protocols, resource constraints, and clinician hesitancy to perform invasive procedures early in critical illness.[23]

It is important to underscore that the combined approach is not universally indicated. Patients with rapidly resolving pneumonia, severe coagulopathy, or poor prognostic indicators (e.g., multiorgan failure or do-not-intubate orders), may not derive benefit from either procedure. Clinical judgment, supported by validated severity scores and multidisciplinary input, is essential to tailor procedural timing and ensure optimal outcomes.[24]

6.5 Conclusion

In patients with severe community-acquired pneumonia requiring mechanical ventilation, early bronchoscopy and early tracheostomy are two procedural interventions that can significantly impact clinical outcomes. Bronchoscopy performed within 72 hours enables airway clearance and enhances microbial diagnosis, while tracheostomy within 7 days facilitates pulmonary hygiene, reduces ventilator-associated complications, and accelerates weaning.

When used in combination, these interventions may provide synergistic benefit by improving respiratory physiology and streamlining critical care management. However, these procedures are not without risk, and must be approached with careful patient selection and institutional readiness. Future randomized controlled trials are needed to clarify optimal timing, identify patient subgroups most likely to benefit, and establish integrated protocols for early procedural interventions in sCAP.

References

1. Tran QK, Nguyen MT, et al. Early tracheostomy in critically ill patients with severe community-acquired pneumonia: Impact on clinical outcomes. *Respir Med.* 2022;191:106715.

2. Lee J, Kim Y, Park S, et al. Impact of early bronchoscopy on outcomes in patients with severe pneumonia requiring mechanical ventilation. *Crit Care.* 2020;24(1):123.

3. Zhang L, Wang X, Liu Y, et al. Association of early bronchoscopy with clinical outcomes in critically ill patients with pneumonia: A retrospective cohort study using MIMIC-IV database. *Ann Intensive Care.* 2023;13(1):56.

4. Kalil AC, Metersky ML, Klompas M, et al. Management of adults with hospital-acquired and ventilator-associated pneumonia: 2016 clinical practice guidelines. *Clin Infect Dis.* 2016;63(5):e61–e111.

5. Hassan M, El-Fattah M, Mousa A, et al. Early bronchoscopy in mechanically ventilated patients with aspiration pneumonitis: A randomized controlled trial. *Egypt J Crit Care Med.* 2021;9(2):45–52.

6. Zhang L, Sun W, Wang Y, et al. The effect of early bronchoscopy on mechanically ventilated patients with pneumonia: A propensity score-matched study. *BMC Pulm Med.* 2021;21:84.

7. Zhang X, Xu X, Zhang Y, et al. Early bronchoscopy improves outcomes in patients with ventilator-associated pneumonia: A single-center study. *J Thorac Dis.* 2022;14(5):1470–1478.

8. Ahn C, Park Y, Oh Y. Early bronchoscopy in severe pneumonia patients in intensive care unit: insights from the MIMIC-IV database analysis. *Acute Crit Care.* 2024;39(1):66–76.

9. Damas P, Frippiat F, Ancion A, et al. Diagnostic yield of fiberoptic bronchoscopy in the intensive care unit: A prospective observational study. *Ann Intensive Care.* 2022;12(1):49.

10. Heininger A, Braun J, Ruesseler M, et al. Risk and safety profile of fiberoptic bronchoscopy in the ICU: A prospective observational study. *Respir Med.* 2020;169:106020.

11. Trouillet JL, Luyt CE, Guiguet M, et al. Early percutaneous tracheotomy versus prolonged intubation in ICU patients: A randomized trial. *JAMA.* 2006;291(20):2540–2547.

12. Griffiths J, Barber VS, Morgan L, Young JD. Systematic review and meta-analysis of studies of the timing of tracheostomy in adult patients undergoing artificial ventilation. *BMJ.* 2005;330(7502):1243.

13. Hosokawa K, Nishimura M, Egi M, Vincent JL. Timing of tracheotomy in ICU patients: A systematic review of randomized controlled trials. *Crit Care.* 2015;19:424.
14. Andriolo BN, Andriolo RB, Saconato H, Atallah ÁN, Valente O. Early versus late tracheostomy for critically ill patients. *Cochrane Database Syst Rev.* 2015;(1):CD007271.
15. Rumbak MJ, Newton M, Truncale T, Schwartz SW, Adams JW, Hazard PB. A prospective, randomized, study comparing early percutaneous tracheostomy to prolonged translaryngeal intubation. *Chest.* 2004;126(1):211–215.
16. Smith RB, et al. Safety and outcomes of percutaneous dilatational versus surgical tracheostomy: A meta-analysis. *Crit Care Med.* 2020;48(3):e250–e257.
17. Nguyen HT, et al. Comparative outcomes of percutaneous and surgical tracheostomy in severe pneumonia patients. *J Thorac Dis.* 2021;13(11):6370–6378.
18. Vargas M, Servillo G, Arditi E, et al. Early percutaneous tracheostomy in patients with moderate to severe acute respiratory distress syndrome. *Respir Care.* 2015;60(10):1436–1441.
19. Scales DC, Thiruchelvam D, Kiss A, Redelmeier DA. The effect of tracheostomy timing during critical illness on long-term survival. *Crit Care Med.* 2008;36(9):2547–2557.
20. Mahmood K, Wahidi MM. The role of bronchoscopy in pneumonia. *Clin Chest Med.* 2018;39(1):155–165.
21. Lee CH, Huang YT, Shih CM, et al. Impact of early bronchoscopy and tracheostomy on critically ill pneumonia patients: A nationwide cohort study. *Respir Investig.* 2021;59(1):53–61.
22. Zhou F, Yu T, Du R, et al. Clinical course and risk factors for mortality in adult inpatients with COVID-19 in Wuhan, China: A retrospective cohort study. *Lancet.* 2020;395(10229):1054–1062.
23. Dondorp AM, Hayat M, Aryal D, Beane A, Schultz MJ. Respiratory support in COVID-19 patients, with a focus on resource-limited settings. *Am J Trop Med Hyg.* 2020;102(6):1191–1197.
24. Mehta AB, Syeda SN, Bajpayee L, et al. Factors associated with time to tracheostomy in mechanically ventilated patients and its effect on outcomes. *Crit Care Med.* 2022;50(6):865–874.

CHAPTER 7

Syndromic Testing and Antimicrobial Resistance Genes

7.1 Introduction

Syndromic testing represents an innovative diagnostic method that utilizes multiplex polymerase chain reaction (PCR) to detect various respiratory pathogens and resistance markers from a single specimen, offering results within hours. This approach has emerged in response to the limitations of conventional diagnostics, which often rely on sequential, pathogen-specific testing and time-consuming culture methods.

Conventional culture, serology, and antigen-based techniques may take 24–72 hours or longer to yield results and are often limited in their ability to detect fastidious or non-culturable organisms. In contrast, syndromic testing enables rapid, comprehensive, and simultaneous detection of multiple pathogens and resistance genes, providing actionable information early in the clinical course.[1,2]

DOI:10.1201/9781003629504-7

7.2 Limitations of Conventional Diagnostic Methods

Traditional diagnostic techniques, including culture, serology, and antigen-based tests, often fall short in detecting polymicrobial infections, atypical bacteria, and slow-growing or fastidious organisms. Conventional cultures may take 48 to 72 hours—or longer—to yield results, and, in some cases, pathogens such as *Legionella pneumophila, Mycoplasma pneumoniae,* and *Chlamydia pneumoniae* are entirely missed due to their fastidious nature or lack of cell wall structure, which hinders growth on standard media.[3,4] Moreover, viral and fungal pathogens are notoriously difficult to detect using traditional methods unless specific suspicion and targeted testing are pursued.

These limitations are further amplified in critically ill patients, where delays in initiating appropriate antimicrobial therapy significantly increase morbidity and mortality. For example, studies have shown that each hour of delay in administering appropriate antibiotics in septic shock is associated with a measurable increase in mortality risk.[5] Additionally, traditional methods lack sensitivity in the presence of prior antibiotic exposure, which is common in hospitalized patients. This underscores an urgent clinical need for faster, broader, and more reliable diagnostic modalities that can support early and precise treatment decisions.

7.3 Principles of Syndromic Testing

Syndromic assays employ multiplex polymerase chain reaction (PCR) technology to simultaneously detect a broad array of respiratory pathogens—including common bacteria, atypical organisms, viruses, and key antimicrobial resistance (AMR) genes—from a single clinical specimen. Respiratory samples such as bronchoalveolar lavage (BAL), endotracheal aspirates (ETA), and sputum are commonly used, although upper airway specimens may be appropriate in selected clinical scenarios.[1,6] These assays typically deliver results within 1 to 6 hours, providing a substantial improvement over conventional diagnostic turnaround times.

Most currently available commercial platforms can detect over 20 respiratory pathogens and more than 10 AMR markers in a single run. The comprehensive scope of syndromic panels supports early, targeted antimicrobial decision-making, reduces reliance on broad-spectrum empiric therapy, and enhances infection control interventions. These tools are particularly beneficial in critically ill or immunocompromised patients, where early and precise pathogen identification is essential for optimal outcomes.[7–9]

7.4 Pathogen Detection in Community-Acquired Pneumonia

Beyond rapid qualitative detection, syndromic panels increasingly offer semi-quantitative data, which introduces a new dimension in clinical interpretation. Importantly, syndromic panels not only provide qualitative identification but also offer semi-quantitative results, expressed as copies per milliliter. These quantitative thresholds can inform clinical interpretation, particularly in distinguishing colonization from true infection. For instance, thresholds of $\geq 10^4$ copies/mL in bronchoalveolar lavage (BAL) and $\geq 10^5$ copies/mL in endotracheal aspirates (ETA) have been suggested to correlate with clinically significant infection rather than colonization.[10]

Several studies have demonstrated that higher bacterial loads, particularly $>10^7$ copies/mL, are associated with more severe disease, greater systemic inflammation, and longer hospital stays. Therefore, quantitative data should be interpreted alongside clinical signs (fever, leukocytosis, radiographic findings) to guide therapy decisions.[11]

In adult patients with community-acquired pneumonia (CAP), syndromic assays enhance the detection of common bacterial pathogens such as *Streptococcus pneumoniae*, *Haemophilus influenzae*, and *Staphylococcus aureus*, as well as atypical bacteria, including *Mycoplasma pneumoniae*, *Legionella pneumophila*, and *Chlamydia pneumoniae*. Viral pathogens such as respiratory syncytial virus (RSV), influenza viruses, and SARS-CoV-2 are also readily detected.[1,12]

This broad pathogen coverage allows for early and precise treatment decisions, reducing delays and minimizing unnecessary use of broad-spectrum antibiotics.

Syndromic testing is especially beneficial in detecting polymicrobial infections, which are common in elderly patients, those with chronic lung disease, or individuals receiving immunosuppressive therapy. Mixed infections involving both viral and bacterial pathogens—such as Influenza A with *Streptococcus pneumoniae*—can worsen disease severity and are often underdiagnosed with conventional methods.[13] Furthermore, in immunocompromised hosts, rapid identification of uncommon pathogens (e.g., human metapneumovirus, *Chlamydia pneumoniae*) may significantly impact early therapeutic decisions and isolation precautions.[14]

7.5 Detection of Antimicrobial Resistance Genes

The presence of resistance genes detected by molecular methods does not always correlate with phenotypic resistance. This discrepancy can arise due to gene silencing, incomplete gene expression, or the presence of nonfunctional gene variants.[15,16] For example, mecA-positive *Staphylococcus aureus* may remain susceptible to oxacillin in rare cases due to regulatory gene mutations or suppressed expression.

Therefore, while the detection of genes such as bla_KPC or bla_NDM signals a high likelihood of resistance, definitive treatment should be based on phenotypic susceptibility results when available. Clinicians are advised to interpret genotypic resistance in the context of the pathogen, specimen source, and patient risk factors. Beyond pathogen identification, syndromic panels provide crucial data on antimicrobial resistance genes. This is particularly important in healthcare-associated pneumonia and infections involving multidrug-resistant organisms (MDROs) (Table 7.1). Common resistance genes detected include:

■ bla_KPC, bla_NDM, and bla_OXA-48: Encode carbapenemases that hydrolyze carbapenem antibiotics.
■ mecA and mecC: Confer methicillin resistance in *Staphylococcus aureus.*
■ The bla prefix denotes genes producing β-lactamase enzymes that inactivate β-lactam antibiotics.[17,18]

Table 7.1 Common Syndromic Testing Panels for Severe Pneumonia and Related Infections

Syndrome/ Condition	Pathogens Detected (Approx.)	Turnaround Time	Key Features
Pneumonia (HAP/ VAP)	>30 pathogens + resistance genes	1 hour	Includes semi-quantitative reporting and AMR genes like blaKPC, blaNDM
Respiratory Infections	>20 pathogens	1 hour	Viral, bacterial, atypical pathogens; includes resistance markers like mecA
	22 pathogens	1 hour	Suitable for point-of-care; rapid results

(*Continued*)

Table 7.1 (Continued)

Syndrome/ Condition	Pathogens Detected (Approx.)	Turnaround Time	Key Features
Gastrointestinal Infections	22 pathogens	1 hour	Covers viral, bacterial, and parasitic GI pathogens
	15 pathogens	5–6 hours	Stool-based multiplex PCR platform
Meningitis/ Encephalitis	14 pathogens	1 hour	Detects both viral and bacterial CNS infections
Bloodstream Infections	43 targets	1 hour	Detects Gram-positive, Gram-negative, yeast, and resistance genes
Sexually Transmitted Infections	3 pathogens	3 hours	High sensitivity and FDA-approved
	2 pathogens	90 minutes	Real-time PCR for Chlamydia and Gonorrhea

Abbreviations: HAP: Hospital-Acquired Pneumonia, VAP: Ventilator-Associated Pneumonia, AMR: Antimicrobial Resistance, PCR: Polymerase Chain Reaction, GI: Gastrointestinal, CNS: Central Nervous System, FDA: Food and Drug Administration, blaKPC: Beta-lactamase *Klebsiella pneumoniae* carbapenemase, blaNDM: Beta-lactamase New Delhi metallo-beta-lactamase, mecA: Gene encoding methicillin resistance in *Staphylococcus aureus*

7.6 Clinical Relevance and Impact on Outcomes

A recent study by Singh et al. highlighted the clinical significance of early resistance detection using syndromic diagnostics. The study found that severe pneumonia caused by carbapenem-resistant *Klebsiella pneumoniae*, *Acinetobacter baumannii*, and *Pseudomonas aeruginosa* was associated with increased mortality. Delayed administration of appropriate antibiotic therapy and comorbidities such as renal failure and the need for mechanical ventilation were key contributors to poor outcomes (Figure 7.1).[19]

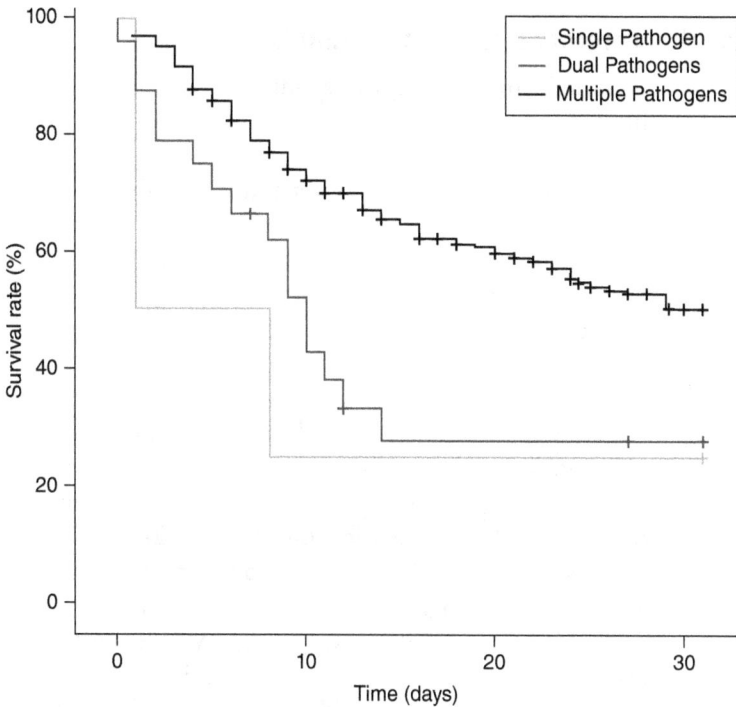

FIGURE 7.1 Kaplan–Meier curve showing survival outcomes in severe pneumonia patients infected with single, dual, and multiple pathogens.[19]

Integrating syndromic test results into clinical decision-making pathways enhances the value of antimicrobial stewardship programs. Hospitals may use these results to create antibiotic de-escalation protocols—for instance, narrowing from broad-spectrum carbapenems to ceftazidime-avibactam in cases with bla_KPC detection.[9] Syndromic testing also plays a critical role in local antibiogram surveillance, allowing infection control teams to map resistance gene prevalence in near real-time.[20] Incorporating molecular results into institutional empirical treatment guidelines, particularly for high-risk units (ICU, oncology, transplant), can promote rational antibiotic use and reduce resistance pressure.

7.7 Interpretation Challenges and Limitations

Despite its many strengths, syndromic testing has several limitations:

■ Detection of resistance genes does not always equate to phenotypic resistance.

■ Pathogen detection may reflect colonization rather than active infection, especially in patients with chronic respiratory conditions.

To address this, clinical interpretation should be integrated with traditional culture and susceptibility testing. Quantitative thresholds, such as $\geq 10^4$ copies/mL for BAL samples and $\geq 10^5$ copies/mL for ETA, help distinguish colonization from true infection (Figure 7.2).[21]

These operational strengths, however, must be balanced against logistical and financial realities, particularly in resource-limited settings. While syndromic testing platforms offer substantial clinical advantages, implementation must consider resource availability and cost-effectiveness. Several health economic studies have suggested that upfront costs associated with syndromic panels are offset by reduced ICU stay, faster targeted therapy, and fewer adverse drug reactions.[12,22] In low- and middle-income countries (LMICs), however, affordability and sustainability remain key challenges. Adopting syndromic testing in these settings may require selective use criteria (e.g., ICU admissions, non-resolving pneumonia) and support from national laboratory networks. Cost–benefit modeling tailored to local resistance patterns is essential to guide policymaker investment.

A potential pitfall of syndromic testing is overdiagnosis, particularly when colonizing organisms are detected in the absence of clear clinical infection. For example, *Haemophilus influenzae* and *Staphylococcus aureus* are known colonizers in patients with chronic obstructive pulmonary disease (COPD) or bronchiectasis. Treating

Result Summary

Bacteria

	Bin (copies/mL)		Bin (copies/mL)			
			10^4	10^5	10^6	≥10^7
Not Detected		*Acinetobacter calcoaceticus-baumannii* complex				
Not Detected		*Enterobacter cloacae* complex				
✓ Detected	≥10^7	*Escherichia coli*	////	////	////	////
Not Detected		*Haemophilus influenzae*				
Not Detected		*Klebsiella aerogenes*				
Not Detected		*Klebsiella oxytoca*				
✓ Detected	≥10^7	*Klebsiella pneumoniae* group	////	////	////	////
Not Detected		*Moraxella catarrhalis*				
Not Detected		*Proteus* spp.				
Not Detected		*Pseudomonas aeruginosa*				
Not Detected		*Serratia marcescens*				
Not Detected		*Staphylococcus aureus*				
Not Detected		*Streptococcus agalactiae*				
Not Detected		*Streptococcus pneumoniae*				
Not Detected		*Streptococcus pyogenes*				

⚠ Note: Detection of bacterial nucleic acid may be indicative of colonizing or normal respiratory flora and may not indicate the causative agent of pneumonia. Semi-quantitative Bin (copies/mL) results generated by the FilmArray Pneumonia Panel *plus* are not equivalent to CFU/mL and do not consistently correlate with the quantity of bacterial analytes compared to CFU/mL. For specimens with multiple bacteria detected, the relative abundance of nucleic acids (copies/mL) may not correlate with the relative abundance of bacteria as determined by culture (CFU/mL). Clinical correlation is advised to determine significance of semi-quantitative Bin (copies/mL) for clinical management.

Antimicrobial Resistance Genes

✓ Detected	CTX-M
Not Detected	IMP
Not Detected	KPC
⊘ N/A	*mecA/C* and MREJ
✓ Detected	NDM
Not Detected	OXA-48-like
Not Detected	VIM

⚠ Note: Antimicrobial resistance can occur via multiple mechanisms. A Not Detected result for a genetic marker of antimicrobial resistance does not indicate susceptibility to associated antimicrobial drugs or drug classes. A Detected result for a genetic marker of antimicrobial resistance cannot be definitively linked to the microorganism(s) detected. Culture is required to obtain isolates for antimicrobial susceptibility testing and FilmArray Pneumonia Panel *plus* results should be used in conjunction with culture results for the determination of susceptibility or resistance.

Atypical Bacteria

Not Detected	*Chlamydia pneumoniae*
Not Detected	*Legionella pneumophila*
Not Detected	*Mycoplasma pneumoniae*

Viruses

Not Detected	Adenovirus
Not Detected	Coronavirus
Not Detected	Human Metapneumovirus
✓ Detected	Human Rhinovirus/Enterovirus
Not Detected	Influenza A
Not Detected	Influenza B
Not Detected	Middle East Respiratory Syndrome Coronavirus (MERS-CoV)
Not Detected	Parainfluenza Virus
✓ Detected	Respiratory Syncytial Virus

FIGURE 7.2 Example of a syndromic test result using the Pneumonia Panel, showing detection of *Klebsiella pneumoniae* (≥10^7 copies/mL), CTX-M resistance gene, and co-infection with Influenza A, Human Rhinovirus/Enterovirus, and RSV.

all positive results without clinical correlation can lead to overtreatment, antibiotic resistance, and unnecessary patient harm.[6]

As such, clinicians should apply antimicrobial stewardship principles, evaluating whether positive results align with symptoms, radiologic evidence, and host immune status. Negative predictive value may be more actionable in ruling out infection than positive results in certain contexts.

7.8 Surveillance and Antimicrobial Stewardship

The rise in antimicrobial resistance underscores the importance of syndromic testing in surveillance and stewardship. The PROTEKT US study documented increasing rates of macrolide-resistant *S. pneumoniae*, highlighting the need for rapid resistance detection to guide empirical therapy and minimize inappropriate antibiotic use.[22] As molecular diagnostics evolve, their integration with digital technologies opens new frontiers in personalized and predictive pneumonia management. Emerging technologies are integrating syndromic testing data with machine learning algorithms to assist in diagnosis, prognostication, and antibiotic selection. Platforms that combine real-time PCR data, patient vitals, laboratory biomarkers, and imaging findings have shown promise in predicting outcomes such as ICU admission, mechanical ventilation, and mortality.[23]

Future research should focus on leveraging artificial intelligence (AI) to optimize the clinical interpretation of syndromic test results and incorporate them into electronic clinical decision support systems (CDSS), particularly in resource-constrained settings where expert infectious disease consultation may not be readily available.

7.9 Conclusion

Syndromic diagnostic platforms are a valuable advancement in the management of severe pneumonia. By enabling rapid and precise identification of respiratory pathogens and resistance genes, these technologies support early and appropriate treatment decisions, reduce antimicrobial misuse, and improve patient outcomes. However, their utility is maximized when used in conjunction with clinical evaluation, phenotypic testing, and local resistance surveillance.[2,19]

References

1. Babady NE. The FilmArray respiratory panel: an automated, broadly multiplexed molecular test for the rapid and accurate detection of respiratory pathogens. *Expert Rev Mol Diagn.* 2013;13(8):779–788.
2. Ginocchio CC, McAdam AJ. Current best practices for respiratory virus testing. *J Clin Microbiol.* 2011;49(9 Suppl):S44–S48.
3. Waites KB, Talkington DF. Mycoplasma pneumoniae and its role as a human pathogen. *Clin Microbiol Rev.* 2004;17(4):697–728.
4. Mandell LA, Wunderink RG, Anzueto A, et al. Infectious Diseases Society of America/American Thoracic Society consensus guidelines on the management of community-acquired pneumonia in adults. *Clin Infect Dis.* 2007;44 Suppl 2:S27–S72.
5. Kumar A, Roberts D, Wood KE, et al. Duration of hypotension before initiation of effective antimicrobial therapy is the critical determinant of survival in human septic shock. *Crit Care Med.* 2006;34(6):1589–1596.
6. Ramanan P, Bryson AL, Binnicker MJ, Pritt BS, Patel R. Syndromic panel-based testing in clinical microbiology. *Clin Microbiol Revi.* 2018;31(1):e00024–e00017. doi:10.1128/CMR.00024-17

7. Beal SG, Thomas C. Practical implementation of respiratory panel testing in the hospital setting. *Diagn Microbiol Infect Dis.* 2017;89(3):162–167. doi:10.1016/j.diagmicrobio.2017.08.013

8. Leber AL, Everhart K, Balada-Llasat JM, et al. Multicenter evaluation of a multiplex molecular panel for detection of bacterial and viral pathogens and antimicrobial resistance genes in lower respiratory tract specimens. *J Clin Microbiol.* 2018;56(6):e01945-17. doi:10.1128/JCM.01945-17.

9. Timbrook TT, Morton JB, McConeghy KW, Caffrey AR, Mylonakis E, LaPlante KL. The effect of molecular rapid diagnostic testing on clinical outcomes in bloodstream infections: a systematic review and meta-analysis. *Clin Infect Dis.* 2017;64(1):15–23. doi:10.1093/cid/ciw649

10. Han JH, Sullivan N, Leas BF, Pegues DA, Kaczmarek JL, Umscheid CA. Impact of multiplex PCR respiratory pathogen testing on clinical outcomes: a systematic review and meta-analysis. *Clin Infect Dis.* 2020;71(9):2134–2140.

11. Rogers BB, Shankar P, Jerris RC, et al. Impact of a rapid respiratory panel test on patient outcomes. *Arch Pathol Lab Med.* 2015;139(5):636–641.

12. Brendish NJ, Malachira AK, Armstrong L, et al. Routine molecular point-of-care testing for respiratory viruses in adults presenting to hospital with acute respiratory illness (ResPOC): a pragmatic, open-label, randomised controlled trial. *Lancet Respir Med.* 2017;5(5):401–411.

13. Moreno G, Rodríguez A, Reyes LF, et al. Severe co-infections in critically ill patients with influenza pneumonia: incidence, etiology and outcomes. *Crit Care.* 2020;24:605.

14. Gaydos CA. What do we know about mixed respiratory infections? *Diagn Microbiol Infect Dis.* 2020;96(4):114949.

15. van Belkum A, Dunne WM Jr. Next-generation antimicrobial susceptibility testing. *J Clin Microbiol.* 2013;51(7):2018–2024.

16. Croxen MA, Lee TD, Hoang LMN. Molecular and phenotypic diagnostics for antimicrobial resistance: a review. *Clin Microbiol Rev.* 2023;36(1):e00151-22.

17. Nordmann P, Naas T, Poirel L. Global spread of Carbapenemase-producing Enterobacteriaceae. *Emerg Infect Dis.* 2011;17(10):1791–1798.

18. Chambers HF. Methicillin resistance in staphylococci: molecular and biochemical basis and clinical implications. *Clin Microbiol Rev.* 1997;10(4):781–791.

19. Singh G, et al. Factors associated with antibiotic resistance and survival analysis of severe pneumonia patients infected with *Klebsiella pneumoniae, Acinetobacter baumannii,* and *Pseudomonas aeruginosa*: a retrospective cohort study in Jakarta, Indonesia. *J Infect Public Health.* 2024. doi:10.1177/20503121241264097

20. Buehler SS, Madison B, Snyder SR, et al. Effectiveness and cost-effectiveness of multiplex nucleic acid amplification tests for diagnosis of respiratory infections: A systematic review and meta-analysis. *Clin Infect Dis.* 2019;68(3):430–440.

21. Ramirez JA, et al. Etiology of community-acquired pneumonia in hospitalized patients in the United States: Results from the Pneumonia Patient Outcomes Research Team (PORT) cohort study. *Clin Infect Dis.* 1999;29(3):447–456.

22. Farrell DJ, et al. Increased antimicrobial resistance among respiratory tract pathogens from US medical centers: results from the PROTEKT US surveillance study, 2000–2003. *J Antimicrob Chemother.* 2004;53(6):1076–1084.

23. Topol EJ. High-performance medicine: the convergence of human and artificial intelligence. *Nat Med.* 2019;25(1):44–56.

CHAPTER 8

Severe Pneumonia in Tropical Infections and Immunocompromised Host

8.1 Introduction

Severe pneumonia occurring in tropical regions is frequently linked to endemic pathogens.[1] Among these, *Burkholderia pseudomallei*, responsible for melioidosis, stands out.[2] This bacterium is prevalent in soil and stagnant water across Southeast Asia and Northern Australia and can induce fatal pneumonia and septicemia, especially in individuals with underlying health conditions or occupational exposure.[1,2]

8.2 Bacterial Etiologies

In tropical regions, bacterial infections play a crucial role in the development of severe pneumonia.[1] Among these, *Mycobacterium tuberculosis* remains a leading cause, often presenting as community-acquired or hospital-associated pneumonia, especially in areas where the disease is endemic.[3] Its radiological findings are frequently nonspecific, which can delay diagnosis. *Burkholderia*

 DOI:10.1201/9781003629504-8

pseudomallei, the pathogen responsible for melioidosis, is another important agent in tropical climates, while *Leptospira* spp., typically transmitted through contact with water contaminated by animal urine, can lead to life-threatening pulmonary complications such as hemorrhage and acute respiratory distress syndrome (ARDS).[2] Furthermore, *Streptococcus pneumoniae* and *Klebsiella pneumoniae* are frequently isolated in patients from low- and middle-income tropical countries and are associated with high morbidity and mortality, particularly in individuals with delayed access to medical care or pre-existing health conditions.[1-3]

From an epidemiological perspective, the highest burden of severe bacterial pneumonia is observed in regions such as Southeast Asia, sub-Saharan Africa, and parts of Latin America. Populations with underlying respiratory conditions are especially vulnerable.[1] This includes individuals with structural lung abnormalities such as chronic obstructive pulmonary disease (COPD), post-tuberculosis lung disease, bronchiectasis, or chronic fungal infections like pulmonary aspergillosis, as well as those with lung malignancies. These conditions compromise lung defenses, increasing the risk of severe infection and poor clinical outcomes.[3-5]

8.3 Viral Etiologies

Viral infections are increasingly recognized as significant contributors to severe pneumonia in tropical settings. Arboviruses such as dengue, chikungunya, and Zika virus can lead to respiratory complications through either direct pulmonary involvement or secondary bacterial infections. The emergence of novel respiratory viruses—including influenza A (H_1N_1), Middle East respiratory syndrome coronavirus (MERS-CoV), and more recently, SARS-CoV-2—has further highlighted the vulnerability of tropical and resource-limited populations to epidemic and pandemic threats. During the 2009 H_1N_1 pandemic, South Korea experienced a significant burden of severe cases, many requiring intensive care and mechanical ventilation, particularly among individuals with underlying respiratory and metabolic conditions. In the Middle East, MERS-CoV has remained endemic since its emergence in 2012, with recurrent outbreaks reported in Saudi Arabia, often linked to zoonotic transmission and nosocomial spread. The COVID-19 pandemic, caused by SARS-CoV-2, had a profound global impact, with disproportionate mortality observed in patients with pre-existing lung diseases.[6,7] A study by Singh et al. demonstrated that low counts of CD4+ T-cells in bronchoalveolar lavage fluid were associated with higher rates of extubation failure and mortality in critically ill COVID-19 pneumonia patients, underscoring the importance of local immune responses in disease progression.[8,9] These viral pneumonias can progress rapidly to ARDS, often necessitating advanced respiratory support that is frequently inaccessible in rural or under-resourced areas.[6–8]

8.4 Fungal and Parasitic Etiologies

Fungal and parasitic infections represent critical etiologies of pneumonia in tropical regions, particularly among immunocompromised hosts. *Histoplasma capsulatum*, endemic in parts of Central and South America, can cause severe disseminated disease with pulmonary involvement in individuals with advanced immunosuppression. According to a case described by Singh in *Challenging Cases in Respirology and Critical Care*, disseminated histoplasmosis may present with prolonged fever and respiratory symptoms, often mimicking tuberculosis. The risk of such dissemination is markedly increased when CD4 counts fall below 150 cells/mm^3, and especially below 50 cells/mm^3 (Figure 8.1).[12] Similarly, *Talaromyces marneffei*, prevalent in Southeast Asia, can lead to severe pulmonary

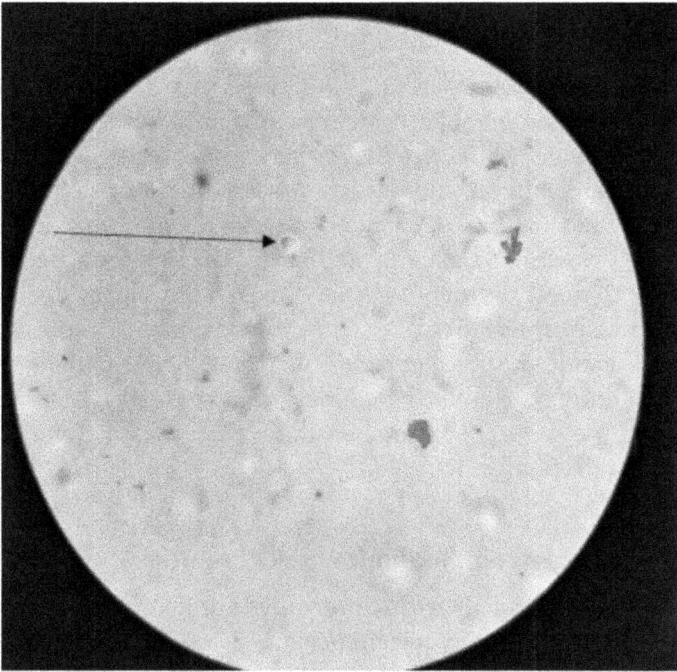

FIGURE 8.1 Histoplasma capsulatum yeast element found in the patient's bone marrow puncture (BMP) specimen (arrow). The specimen was visualized using Wright–Giemsa staining. (Magnification: 1000x)

disease in patients with HIV/AIDS or other forms of immune suppression.[10–11] *Pneumocystis jirovecii* pneumonia (PJP) remains a common opportunistic infection in individuals with HIV infection, particularly when CD4 counts are below 200 cells/mm³. Parasitic infections such as *Plasmodium falciparum* can produce severe malaria with respiratory complications, including non-cardiogenic pulmonary edema and ARDS. Moreover, *Strongyloides stercoralis* hyperinfection may lead to fatal pneumonia in patients receiving corticosteroids or other forms of immunosuppressive therapy.

8.5 Role of Climate Change

The rising prevalence and spread of tropical infectious diseases have been significantly influenced by climate change. Shifts in climate parameters such as temperature, rainfall, and humidity affect the habitats of vectors like mosquitoes, enabling the expansion of illnesses like dengue and malaria into areas previously unaffected.[4] Natural disasters such as floods and cyclones can also impair healthcare systems, increase human crowding, and lead to greater exposure to waterborne and airborne pathogens. These conditions heighten the risk of secondary bacterial pneumonia and other serious respiratory infections.[5]

8.6 Severe Pneumonia in Immunocompromised Hosts

In individuals with compromised immune systems, the causes of severe pneumonia are diverse and often involve opportunistic pathogens. Viruses such as cytomegalovirus (CMV), respiratory syncytial virus (RSV), influenza, adenovirus, and SARS-CoV-2 frequently cause severe disease with high mortality rates in this group.[13] CMV reactivation is increasingly recognized as a significant cause of pneumonia in non-HIV immunocompromised patients, including those undergoing immunosuppressive therapy or critical illness. CMV pneumonia is often challenging to diagnose due to nonspecific clinical and radiological findings but can lead to severe respiratory failure if untreated. Early recognition and antiviral therapy are crucial to improve outcomes.[14]

Opportunistic fungi, including *Pneumocystis jirovecii*, *Aspergillus* species, and *Cryptococcus* species, are major concerns in patients with neutropenia or defective cell-mediated immunity, such as those undergoing chemotherapy or receiving organ transplants.[10–12] Additionally, bacteria such as *Pseudomonas aeruginosa* and *Staphylococcus aureus* are prevalent among hospitalized or mechanically ventilated patients. Tuberculosis continues to be a major contributor to pulmonary complications in immunocompromised individuals, particularly in people with HIV, often presenting with atypical features that complicate diagnosis. Beyond *Mycobacterium tuberculosis*, Non-Tuberculous Mycobacteria (NTM), such as *Mycobacterium avium* complex and *Mycobacterium abscessus*, are increasingly recognized as opportunistic pathogens, especially in patients with underlying lung disease or immunosuppression. These infections may mimic TB clinically and radiologically but require different therapeutic approaches, as summarized in (Table 8.1).[15–17]

TABLE 8.1 Common Pathogens Causing Severe Pneumonia in Immunocompromised Hosts

Type	Common Pathogens	At-Risk Populations
Bacteria	*Streptococcus pneumoniae, Staphylococcus aureus, Pseudomonas aeruginosa, Klebsiella pneumoniae, Haemophilus influenzae, Acinetobacter baumannii*	Hospitalized patients, ventilated patients, neutropenic patients, elderly, organ transplant recipients
Atypical bacteria	*Legionella pneumophila, Mycoplasma pneumoniae, Chlamydophila pneumoniae*	Immunocompromised, cancer patients, those receiving immunosuppressive therapy
Viruses	Influenza A/B, respiratory syncytial virus (RSV), cytomegalovirus (CMV), SARS-CoV-2	Transplant recipients, HIV/AIDS, hematologic malignancies

(Continued)

TABLE 8.1 (Continued)

Type	Common Pathogens	At-Risk Populations
Fungi	*Aspergillus* spp., *Pneumocystis jirovecii, Cryptococcus* spp.	HIV/AIDS, neutropenic patients, patients on long-term corticosteroids or chemotherapy
Mycobacterium tuberculosis	*Mycobacterium tuberculosis*	HIV-positive individuals, patients from TB-endemic regions, immunosuppressed patients
Nontuberculous mycobacteria	*Mycobacterium avium* complex, *M. abscessus, M. kansasii*	Structural lung disease (e.g., bronchiectasis, COPD), elderly, immunocompromised

8.7 Pathogenesis

The pathogenesis of severe pneumonia in immunocompromised hosts involves both host- and pathogen-related factors. Immunosuppression impairs mucosal barriers and innate immune defenses, facilitating microbial invasion and colonization of the lower respiratory tract.[8,9] Deficiencies in neutrophil function, macrophage activation, and T-cell-mediated immunity compromise the clearance of pathogens, allowing unchecked proliferation.[8] This can result in diffuse alveolar damage, alveolar filling with exudates, and eventual development of ARDS. For instance, CMV can induce cytopathic effects in alveolar epithelial cells, while invasive aspergillosis leads to tissue necrosis and angioinvasion.[14] Tuberculosis in HIV patients often leads to disseminated or miliary patterns due to an inability to mount a granulomatous response. These pathological processes culminate in severe hypoxemia and respiratory failure, necessitating intensive care interventions.[16]

Moreover, a prospective cohort study by Singh et al. demonstrated that low alveolar macrophage function, low levels of IL-6 in bronchoalveolar lavage fluid (BALF), and high BALF CD4+ cell counts were significantly associated with successful extubation and survival in patients with severe pneumonia. These findings suggest that immune cell profiles and local cytokine environments in the lung contribute to the trajectory of disease in critically ill immunocompromised patients, emphasizing the importance of individualized immunological assessment in the management of severe pneumonia.[8,9]

8.8 Vitamin D and Immune Modulation

Vitamin D has garnered significant attention for its immunomodulatory properties, particularly in the context of respiratory infections among immunocompromised individuals. The active form, 1,25-dihydroxyvitamin D, enhances innate immunity by stimulating the production of antimicrobial peptides such as cathelicidin (LL-37) and defensins, which combat a broad spectrum of pathogens, including bacteria, viruses, and fungi. Moreover, it modulates the immune response by suppressing proinflammatory cytokines like IL-6 and TNF-α, while promoting anti-inflammatory pathways through the activation of regulatory T cells and modulation of dendritic cell activity.[17,18]

Deficiency in vitamin D is prevalent among immunocompromised populations, including individuals with HIV, those undergoing chemotherapy, or transplant recipients, and is associated with an increased risk of severe respiratory infections like pneumonia. Research indicates that insufficient vitamin D levels may impair lung-specific immune responses, leading to heightened susceptibility to microbial colonization and inflammatory damage in pulmonary tissues. Clinical trials and meta-analyses support the role of vitamin D supplementation in reducing the incidence and severity of acute respiratory tract infections, especially among individuals with baseline deficiencies.[19] Regular supplementation, whether daily or weekly, has been shown to significantly lower infection risk, suggesting its potential as a preventive measure in immunocompromised hosts. However, standardized clinical guidelines regarding optimal dosages and target serum levels are still under development, necessitating further research to establish broader clinical efficacy.[16,18]

Beyond vitamin D, other micronutrients, such as vitamins C and E, zinc, and folate, play critical roles in immune function. These nutrients are essential for maintaining the integrity of physical barriers, supporting the proliferation and function of immune cells, and modulating inflammatory responses. Deficiencies in these micronutrients can compromise the immune system, increasing vulnerability to infections. For instance, zinc is vital for the function of various immune cells and has been shown to reduce the duration and severity of respiratory infections when supplemented appropriately. Similarly, vitamin C contributes to immune defense by supporting various cellular functions of both the innate and adaptive immune systems.[17–20]

The gut microbiota also plays a pivotal role in immune modulation. Vitamin D influences the composition and function of the gut microbiome, which in turn affects systemic immunity and the gut–lung axis. A balanced gut microbiota is essential for the development and function of the immune system, and disruptions in this microbial community can lead to dysregulated immune responses and increased susceptibility to respiratory infections. Vitamin D, through its receptor VDR, helps maintain gut microbial homeostasis, thereby contributing to immune resilience.[18,20]

8.9 Conclusion

Severe pneumonia in tropical regions and immunocompromised populations represents a significant clinical and public health challenge, shaped by complex interactions among infectious agents, environmental conditions, and host factors. The diverse etiologies, from endemic bacteria like *Burkholderia pseudomallei* and *Mycobacterium tuberculosis*, to emerging viruses and opportunistic fungal and parasitic pathogens, require context-specific diagnostic and therapeutic strategies. Immunocompromised patients, in particular, face increased susceptibility and worse outcomes, highlighting the need for early identification of at-risk individuals and personalized care approaches. The role of climate change as a driver of disease burden further complicates control efforts, necessitating an integrative, multisectoral response that encompasses environmental management, surveillance, and public health infrastructure strengthening. Meanwhile, evolving evidence on host immune modulators, such as vitamin D, offers promising adjunctive strategies to bolster host defenses in vulnerable populations, though clinical implementation awaits further standardization and consensus.

Future efforts should focus on strengthening region-specific surveillance for emerging pathogens; expanding access to rapid diagnostics and advanced supportive care in low-resource settings; conducting robust clinical trials to evaluate immunomodulatory and adjunctive therapies; and also enhancing interdisciplinary collaboration among infectious disease specialists, pulmonologists, intensivists, and public health experts. Understanding the dynamic landscape of severe pneumonia in tropical and immunocompromised settings is essential to reduce morbidity and mortality. A proactive, evidence-based approach integrating pathogen-specific interventions with host-directed strategies will be critical for improving outcomes in these high-risk populations.

References

1. Meghji J, Mortimer K, Agusti A, Allwood BW, Asher I, Bateman ED, et al. Improving lung health in low-income and middle-income countries: from challenges to solutions. *Lancet.* 2021;397(10277):928–940.

2. Limmathurotsakul D, Golding N, Dance DAB, Messina JP, Pigott DM, Moyes CL, et al. Predicted global distribution of *Burkholderia pseudomallei* and burden of melioidosis. *Nat Microbiol.* 2016;1:15008.

3. World Health Organization. Global tuberculosis report 2023. Geneva: WHO; 2023.

4. Caminade C, McIntyre KM, Jones AE. Impact of recent and future climate change on vector-borne diseases. *Ann N Y Acad Sci.* 2019;1436(1):157–173.

5. Wu X, Lu Y, Zhou S, Chen L, Xu B. Impact of climate change on human infectious diseases: empirical evidence and human adaptation. *Environ Int.* 2016;86:14–23.

6. Choi WS, Lee J, Kim YJ, Kim DW, Lee CH, Ryu SY, et al. Clinical and epidemiological characteristics of the 2009 H1N1 influenza pandemic in South Korea. *Osong Public Health Res Perspect.* 2011;2(1):8–15.

7. Al-Tawfiq JA, Memish ZA. Middle East respiratory syndrome coronavirus: epidemiology and disease control measures. *Infect Drug Resist.* 2020;13:2815–2821.

8. Singh G, Rumende CM, Rengganis I, Amin Z, Loho T, Pranggono EH, Harimurti K, Wibowo H, Fauzi NB, Masse SF, Zakiyah LF. Low alveolar macrophages function, low BALF IL-6 level and high BALF CD4 cell count is associated with successful extubation and survival in severe pneumonia patients: A prospective cohort study. *Indonesia Journal of Chest & Critical Emergency Medicine.* 2024;11(1):3–8.

9. Singh G, Rumende CM, Sharma SK, Rengganis I, Amin Z, Loho T, et al. Low BALF CD4 T cells count is associated with extubation failure and mortality in critically ill COVID-19 pneumonia. *Ann Med.* 2022;54(1):1894–1905.

10. ClinicalInfo HIV.gov. Guidelines for the prevention and treatment of opportunistic infections in adults and adolescents with HIV: Pneumocystis Pneumonia. [Internet]. U.S. Department of Health and Human Services; 2023. Available from: https://clinicalinfo.hiv.gov/en/guidelines/hiv-clinical-guidelines-adult-and-adolescent-opportunistic-infections/pneumocystis

11. Singh G. Disseminated *Histoplasma capsulatum* infection with prolonged fever. In: Singh G, editor. *Challenging Cases in Respirology and Critical Care.* Singapore: Springer; 2025. pp. 149–160.
12. ClinicalInfo HIV.gov. Guidelines for the prevention and treatment of opportunistic infections in adults and adolescents with HIV: Histoplasmosis. [Internet]. U.S. Department of Health and Human Services; 2023. Available from: https://clinicalinfo.hiv.gov/sites/default/files/guidelines/documents/adult-adolescent-oi/histoplasmosis-adult-adolescent-oi.pdf
13. Fishman JA. Infection in solid-organ transplant recipients. *N Engl J Med.* 2007;357(25):2601–2614.
14. Singh G. Reactivation of cytomegalovirus infection in a Non-HIV immunocompromised patient: Case Rreport. *Indones J Chest Med.* 2023;3(4):210–217.
15. Lawn SD, Zumla AI. Tuberculosis. *Lancet.* 2011;378 (9785):57–72.
16. Gupta RK, Lucas SB, Fielding KL, Lawn SD. Prevalence of tuberculosis in post-mortem studies of HIV-infected adults and children in resource-limited settings: a systematic review and meta-analysis. *AIDS.* 2015;29(15): 1987–2002.
17. World Health Organization. Global tuberculosis report 2023. Geneva: WHO; 2023.
18. Aranow C. Vitamin D and the immune system. *J Investig Med.* 2011;59(6):881–886.
19. Martineau AR, Jolliffe DA, Hooper RL, et al. Vitamin D supplementation to prevent acute respiratory infections: systematic review and meta-analysis of individual participant data. *BMJ.* 2017;356:i6583.
20. Hewison M. Vitamin D and the immune system: new perspectives on an old theme. *Endocrinol Metab Clin North Am.* 2010;39(2):365–379.

CHAPTER 9

Non-Infective Pneumonia and Non-Resolving Pneumonia

9.1 Introduction

Pneumonia is classically perceived as an infectious disease; however, a significant subset of patients presents with pneumonia-like symptoms that are not attributable to microbial causes. Non-infective pneumonia encompasses a diverse range of pulmonary inflammatory conditions that mimic bacterial or viral pneumonia both clinically and radiographically, complicating timely diagnosis and appropriate treatment. These include aspiration syndromes, chemical pneumonitis, drug-induced lung injury, vaping-related lung disease, interstitial lung diseases, and immune-mediated pneumonitis. Moreover, non-resolving pneumonia represents another diagnostic and therapeutic challenge, often necessitating re-evaluation for alternative causes such as malignancy, resistant pathogens, pulmonary embolism, or structural lung abnormalities. A thorough understanding of these non-infective and non-resolving presentations is crucial to avoid mismanagement, ensure accurate diagnosis, and implement effective treatment strategies.[1,2]

DOI:10.1201/9781003629504-9

9.2 Non-Infective Pneumonia

Non-infective pneumonia refers to inflammatory conditions of the lung parenchyma without an identifiable microbial etiology. These cases often mimic infectious pneumonia clinically and radiologically, leading to diagnostic delays or mismanagement.[1]

9.2.1 Stroke and Aspiration Pneumonia

Patients with acute stroke are particularly susceptible to aspiration pneumonia due to dysphagia, reduced consciousness, or impaired protective airway reflexes. Early assessment of swallowing function is vital, and Functional Endoscopic Evaluation of Swallowing (FEES) provides direct visualization to guide safe oral intake strategies and feeding support.[1]

9.2.2 Bile Aspiration

Bile acid aspiration, often resulting from gastroesophageal reflux or emesis, can induce chemical pneumonitis. This non-infective inflammatory process may resemble bacterial pneumonia but lacks microbial growth. Persistent inflammation may lead to organizing pneumonia and requires a high index of suspicion.[2]

9.2.3 Drowning and Near-Drowning

Patients who have experienced drowning or near-drowning episodes often present with acute lung injury or non-cardiogenic pulmonary edema. Although initially sterile, aspirated water—especially if contaminated—can cause a severe inflammatory reaction requiring aggressive supportive care and surveillance for secondary infection.[3]

9.2.4 Intravenous Marijuana Use

Although rare, intravenous injection of marijuana oils or extracts has been associated with severe pneumonitis and granulomatous inflammation. Lipid-containing solvents and particulate contamination are thought to mediate the pulmonary injury.[4]

9.2.5 Vaping-Associated Lung Injury

Electronic cigarette or vaping-associated lung injury (EVALI) has emerged as a public health concern. Clinical presentations range from acute eosinophilic or lipoid pneumonia to diffuse alveolar damage. Diagnosis is largely clinical and supported by radiological findings and exclusion of infection. Management involves cessation of exposure and corticosteroid therapy.[5]

9.2.6 Drug-Induced Lung Injury

Drug-induced lung injury (DILI) encompasses a range of pulmonary adverse effects related to pharmaceutical agents. Rituximab, a monoclonal antibody used in hematologic malignancies and autoimmune diseases, has been associated with organizing pneumonia and interstitial pneumonitis. Symptoms often include dry cough, dyspnea, and infiltrates on imaging, which may occur weeks to months after exposure. Statins, commonly used for dyslipidemia, have also been implicated in rare cases of interstitial lung disease and persistent cough. Aspirin, especially in patients with underlying asthma or aspirin-exacerbated respiratory disease (AERD), may cause eosinophilic pneumonitis or bronchospasm. Diagnosis of DILI relies on a thorough temporal drug history, exclusion of infection, and, in some cases, histopathological confirmation. Withdrawal of the offending agent and corticosteroid therapy are commonly required.[6]

9.2.7 Interstitial Lung Disease (ILD)

ILDs are a group of disorders characterized by chronic inflammation and fibrosis of the lung interstitium. Many forms are non-infective in nature and include idiopathic pulmonary fibrosis, connective tissue disease-associated ILD, and hypersensitivity pneumonitis. These conditions often present as chronic dry cough and progressive dyspnea with restrictive patterns on pulmonary function tests and reticular opacities on imaging.[7]

There are various subtypes of interstitial lung diseases (ILDs), each categorized by their underlying causes:

1. Idiopathic Interstitial Pneumonias (IIPs): This category comprises several forms, with idiopathic pulmonary fibrosis (IPF) being the most prevalent and severe. Other types include nonspecific interstitial pneumonia (NSIP), cryptogenic organizing pneumonia (COP), and desquamative interstitial pneumonia (DIP). IPF typically affects older individuals and is associated with poor outcomes, whereas NSIP and COP may respond more favorably to corticosteroids.[8]

2. ILD Associated with Connective Tissue Disorders (CTD-ILD): This form of ILD develops in the context of autoimmune diseases like systemic sclerosis, rheumatoid arthritis, and dermatomyositis. The radiological and pathological features vary but often show a usual interstitial pneumonia (UIP) or NSIP pattern, depending on the specific rheumatologic condition.[9]

3. Hypersensitivity Pneumonitis (HP): Triggered by repeated inhalation of organic antigens such as mold or animal proteins, HP can become chronic and lead to fibrotic changes if not identified early. The disease may initially be reversible but progresses with continued exposure.[10]

4. Environmental and Occupational ILDs: These disorders result from long-term exposure to industrial agents such as asbestos, silica, or coal dust. Conditions like asbestosis, silicosis, and coal workers' pneumoconiosis are preventable and often related to inadequate protective measures in the workplace.[11]

5. Drug- and Radiation-related ILD: Some medications (e.g., methotrexate, bleomycin, amiodarone) and radiation therapy to the thorax can damage lung

tissue. The extent of pulmonary injury depends on the agent used, duration of exposure, and individual sensitivity.[12]

6. Granulomatous ILDs: Sarcoidosis is a primary example of granulomatous interstitial lung disease, typically presenting with non-caseating granuloma formation in the lungs and possibly affecting multiple organ systems such as the skin, eyes, and lymph nodes. The clinical course of sarcoidosis is highly variable, ranging from asymptomatic cases discovered incidentally to progressive disease with multiorgan involvement.[13] A rare variant, necrotizing sarcoid granulomatosis (NSG), has been reported in Indonesia, presenting diagnostic challenges due to its overlap with tuberculosis and malignancy. In a case by Singh et al., a 71-year-old man with prolonged fever and mediastinal lymphadenopathy was initially misdiagnosed with tuberculosis. Diagnosis was confirmed via biopsy showing NSG features, and the patient responded well to corticosteroids. This underscores the importance of clinician awareness and histopathological evaluation in suspected granulomatous lung disease.[14]

Recognizing the ILD subtype is essential for guiding therapy and determining prognosis. Diagnostic assessment usually includes high-resolution CT (HRCT), clinical evaluation, autoimmune serology, and, in some cases, lung biopsy.

9.2.8 Pneumonitis—Allergy-Induced and Immune-Mediated Pneumonia

Pneumonitis refers to non-infective inflammation of the lung parenchyma, typically involving the alveolar walls and interstitium. It can arise from various etiologies, including allergic reactions, drug exposure, radiation, and systemic autoimmune disorders.

One of the most well-characterized forms is Hypersensitivity Pneumonitis (HP), an immunologically mediated condition caused by repeated inhalation of specific antigens such as avian proteins, mold spores, or occupational allergens (e.g., thermophilic actinomycetes in farmers). HP may present in acute, subacute, or chronic forms, with symptoms ranging from episodic cough, dyspnea, and fever to irreversible fibrotic lung disease. Diagnosis hinges on exposure history, HRCT showing centrilobular nodules or mosaic attenuation, and bronchoalveolar lavage with lymphocytosis. Management includes antigen avoidance and corticosteroid therapy in moderate-to-severe cases.[15]

Immune checkpoint inhibitors (ICIs), commonly used in cancer therapy, have been associated with the development of immune-related pneumonitis. Patients typically present with symptoms such as cough, shortness of breath, and new infiltrates on imaging, which may resemble infection or tumor progression. Histopathological examination often reveals features of organizing pneumonia or diffuse alveolar damage. Management involves promptly discontinuing the causative agent and initiating corticosteroid therapy, which remains the mainstay of treatment.[16]

Another important subtype is radiation pneumonitis, typically seen within weeks to months after thoracic radiotherapy, particularly in lung cancer or breast cancer patients. It is characterized by low-grade fever, dry cough, and localized infiltrates on imaging corresponding to the radiation field. Diagnosis is clinical and radiological, and corticosteroid therapy generally leads to improvement.[17]

9.3 Non-Resolving Pneumonia

9.3.1 Definition and Clinical Relevance

Non-resolving pneumonia is characterized by the lack of clinical or radiographic improvement despite appropriate antimicrobial therapy, typically within 72 hours. Persistent symptoms or worsening imaging should prompt consideration of alternative diagnoses.[18]

9.3.2 Re-evaluation After 72 Hours of Therapy

Guidelines recommend reassessing all cases of pneumonia that do not show improvement within three days of treatment. Potential causes include:

- Pulmonary edema, particularly in patients with cardiac disease or fluid overload.
- Pulmonary embolism, presenting with sudden dyspnea or pleuritic chest pain.
- Structural lung abnormalities, including bronchiectasis or obstructive lesions, which hinder antibiotic delivery.
- Alternative infections: *Mycobacterium tuberculosis, Aspergillus, Histoplasma*, and multi-drug resistant (MDR) bacteria should be ruled out.
- Suboptimal antibiotic therapy, including incorrect dosing or administration route, must be reviewed to ensure therapeutic efficacy.[19]

9.3.3 Role of Oral Hygiene

Oral colonization with pathogenic organisms is a common source of persistent pneumonia, particularly in elderly or ventilated patients. Poor oral hygiene contributes to micro-aspiration and prolonged inflammation. Implementing regular oral care, including antiseptic mouthwash and mechanical plaque removal, has been shown to reduce pneumonia incidence and improve outcomes.[20]

9.4 Conclusion

Non-infective and non-resolving pneumonia highlight the complexity of pulmonary medicine, where not all cases of lung inflammation are due to infection. Recognizing alternative etiologies—ranging from aspiration and drug toxicity to autoimmune and environmental factors—is vital in patients who do not respond to conventional antibiotic therapy. For non-resolving pneumonia, timely reassessment after 72 hours of appropriate treatment is essential to avoid delays in identifying more serious underlying causes. Comprehensive evaluation, including imaging, bronchoscopy, and histopathological analysis when necessary, along with attention to modifiable factors such as oral hygiene, can significantly enhance patient outcomes. Ultimately, an individualized and multidisciplinary approach remains key in managing these challenging cases.

References

1. Martino R, Foley N, Bhogal S, Diamant N, Speechley M, Teasell, R. Dysphagia after stroke: Incidence, diagnosis, and pulmonary complications. *Stroke*. 2005;36(12): 2756–2763.
2. Marik PE. Aspiration pneumonitis and aspiration pneumonia. *N Engl J Med*. 2001 Mar;344(9): 665–671.
3. Modell JH, Graves SA. Clinical course of 91 consecutive near-drowning victims. *Chest*. 1976;70(5):631–638.
4. Tashkin DP. Marijuana and lung disease. *Chest*. 2018; 154(3):653–663.
5. Layden JE, Ghinai I, Pray IW, Kimball A, Layer M, Tenforde MW, et al. Pulmonary illness related to e-cigarette use in Illinois and Wisconsin: Preliminary report. *N Engl J Med*. 2020;382(10):903–916.
6. Camus P, Fanton A, Bonniaud P, Camus C, Foucher P. Interstitial lung disease induced by drugs and radiation. *Respiration*. 2004;71(4):301–326.
7. Travis WD, Costabel U, Hansell DM, King TE Jr, Lynch DA, Nicholson AG, et al. An official American Thoracic Society statement: Update of the international multidisciplinary classification of the idiopathic interstitial pneumonias. *Am J Respir Crit Care Med*. 2013;188(6):733–748.
8. Travis WD, Costabel U, Hansell DM, et al. An official American Thoracic Society/European Respiratory society statement: Update of the international multidisciplinary classification of the idiopathic interstitial pneumonias. *Am J Respir Crit Care Med*. 2013;188(6):733–748. doi: 10.1164/rccm.201308-1483ST

9. Fischer A, du Bois R. Interstitial lung disease in connective tissue disorders. *Lancet.* 2012;380(9842):689–698. doi: 10.1016/S0140-6736(12)61079-4

10. Morell F, Villar A, Montero MÁ, Munoz X, Colby TV, Pipvath S, et al. Chronic hypersensitivity pneumonitis in patients diagnosed with idiopathic pulmonary fibrosis: A prospective case-cohort study. *Lancet Respir Med.* 2013;1(9):685–694.

11. DeLight N, Sachs H. Pneumoconiosis. Treasure Publishing; 2025 Jan-[updated 2023 Jul 25]. Available from: https://www.ncbi.nlm.nih.gov/books/NBK555902/

12. Camus P, Fanton A, Bonniaud P, Camus C, Foucher P. Interstitial lung disease induced by drugs and radiation. *Respir Med.* 2004;98(5):459–472. doi: 10.1016/j.rmed.2003.11.003

13. Baughman RP, Valeyre D, Korsten P, Mathioudakis AG, Wuyts WA, Wells A, et al. ERS clinical practice guidelines on treatment of sarcoidosis. *Eur Respir J.* 2021;58(6):2004079.

14. Singh G, Karsono R, Sjamsoe S, Triono MR, Nora RD, Felicia D, Gultom FL, Ruslim D, Sejati A, Gunarsa RG, Pitoyo CW, Rumende CM. Challenges in diagnosing necrotizing sarcoid granulomatosis: The first case reported from Indonesia. *Case Rep Med.* 2025 April 14;2025:3219868. doi: 10.1155/carm/3219868. PMID: 40260189; PMCID: PMC12011462.

15. Selman M, Pardo A, King TE Jr. Hypersensitivity pneumonitis: insights in diagnosis and pathobiology. *Am J Respir Crit Care Med.* 2012;186(4):314–324.

16. Naidoo J, Wang X, Woo KM, Iyriboz T, Halpenny D, Cunningham J, et al. Pneumonitis in patients treated with anti-programmed death-1/programmed death ligand 1 therapy. *J Clin Oncol.* 2017;35(7):709–717.

17. Rodrigues G, Lock M, D'Souza D, Yu E, Van Dyk J. Prediction of radiation pneumonitis by dose–volume histogram parameters in lung cancer: A systematic review. *Radiother Oncol.* 2004;71(2):127–138.

18. Fine MJ, Auble TE, Yealy DM, Hanusa BH, Weissfeld LA, Singer DE, et al. A prediction rule to identify low-risk patients with community-acquired pneumonia. *N Engl J Med.* 1997;336(4):243–250.

19. Metlay JP, Waterer GW, Long AC, Anzueto A, Brozek J, Crothers K, et al. Diagnosis and treatment of adults with community-acquired pneumonia. *Am J Respir Crit Care Med.* 2019;200(7):e45–e67.
20. El-Solh AA, Pietrantoni C, Bhat A, Aquilina A, Okada M, Grover V, et al. Colonization of dental plaques: a reservoir of respiratory pathogens for hospital-acquired pneumonia in institutionalized elders. *Chest.* 2004;126(5):1575–1582.

CHAPTER 10

The Benefits of Palliative Care and Physical Rehabilitation in Patients with Severe Pneumonia

10.1 Introduction

Severe pneumonia often requires hospitalization and intensive care, especially in high-risk individuals. Despite advances in critical care, survivors frequently face prolonged physical and psychological recovery. Symptoms such as dyspnea, fatigue, anxiety, and functional decline are common sequelae. Therefore, attention must be given to strategies beyond pathogen-directed treatment. Palliative care and physical rehabilitation represent two crucial, underutilized components that can improve outcomes in both the acute and post-acute phases of illness.[1,2]

10.2 Palliative Care in Severe Pneumonia

10.2.1 Role and Relevance

Palliative care aims to alleviate suffering through symptom management, psychosocial support, and facilitation

DOI:10.1201/9781003629504-10

of goal-directed care. In severe pneumonia, especially in patients with limited physiological reserve or multiple comorbidities, early palliative involvement can address distressing symptoms like breathlessness and anxiety, support complex decision-making regarding ventilatory support, and enhance communication between care teams and families.[3,4]

10.2.2 Indications for Integration

Palliative care should be considered in patients with advanced age, poor baseline function, multi-organ failure, or underlying terminal illness. These characteristics are often associated with worse outcomes and higher symptom burden, justifying early palliative input to guide the trajectory of care and align it with patient goals.[3]

10.2.3 Common Interventions

Typical interventions include the use of low-dose opioids for dyspnea, benzodiazepines for anxiety, and antipsychotics for delirium management. Additionally, palliative teams facilitate code status discussions, end-of-life planning, and caregiver support, often reducing intensive care unit (ICU) length of stay and unnecessary interventions.[4]

10.3 Physical Rehabilitation in Severe Pneumonia

10.3.1 Importance of Functional Recovery

Patients who survive severe pneumonia often suffer from ICU-acquired weakness, sarcopenia, and cognitive impairment. These issues contribute to prolonged disability and increased healthcare utilization. Physical rehabilitation plays a central role in addressing these complications.[5]

10.3.2 Strategies and Timing

Effective rehabilitation strategies include early mobilization during ICU stay, chest physiotherapy to improve airway clearance, and structured rehabilitation programs post-discharge. Initiating these interventions as early as medically feasible is associated with better recovery of function and reduced complications.[5,6]

Moreover, it is important to emphasize that physical rehabilitation, including ambulation, is feasible even for patients who remain connected to mechanical ventilators, particularly those using portable or transportable ventilators. With careful planning and adequate staffing, ventilated patients can undergo early mobilization and physical therapy, including bedside sitting, transfer to chair, and even ambulation under supervision. Visual documentation of such activities (e.g., photographs of ventilated patients walking with multidisciplinary team support) can be a powerful tool to promote this practice across ICUs.[7,8]

For patients transitioning to home care, particularly those with chronic hypoxemia post-pneumonia, the use of oxygen concentrators plays a pivotal role. These devices provide a stable source of oxygen and support continued recovery, functional independence, and participation in physical rehabilitation programs at home. The integration of home-based rehabilitation and domiciliary oxygen therapy has been shown to improve long-term outcomes in selected survivors of severe pneumonia.[9,10]

10.3.3 Evidence of Benefit

Studies have shown that early physical therapy leads to shorter ICU stay, improved mobility scores, reduced duration of mechanical ventilation, and better long-term quality of life. These benefits are most pronounced when interventions are personalized and started within the ICU.[5,6]

10.4 Integration of Palliative and Rehabilitative Care

10.4.1 Complementary Approaches

Rather than being exclusive, palliative care and rehabilitation complement each other. Palliative care addresses suffering and quality of life, while rehabilitation restores function and independence. Their integration leads to a comprehensive, patient-centered care model in severe pneumonia.[11]

10.4.2 Multidisciplinary Collaboration

Optimal implementation requires collaboration between ICU clinicians, palliative care specialists, rehabilitation therapists, and nursing staff. Evidence supports that early interdisciplinary interventions improve outcomes, reduce readmissions, and align treatments with patient values.[11,12]

A critical, but often under-addressed aspect of multidisciplinary care in patients with severe pneumonia is the integration of advance care planning, including clear documentation and communication regarding code status— specifically Do Not Resuscitate (DNR), Do Not Intubate (DNI), and Do Not Escalate Care (DNC) directives. These designations are essential in ensuring that treatment intensity matches the patient's prognosis, clinical trajectory, and expressed goals of care.[13]

10.4.2.1 Do Not Resuscitate (DNR)

DNR orders indicate that cardiopulmonary resuscitation (CPR) should not be initiated in the event of cardiac arrest. In the context of severe pneumonia, particularly in older adults or those with advanced comorbidities, CPR often has a low likelihood of success and may result in significant suffering. Discussing DNR early, ideally before clinical deterioration, allows families and healthcare teams to prepare for outcomes aligned with the patient's values.[13] However, it is important to note that DNR or Do Not Attempt Resuscitation (DNAR) orders are specific to CPR and do not automatically preclude other intensive treatments, such as vasopressors or mechanical ventilation. For some patients, especially those with a clear end-of-life care plan, vasopressors may also be declined to avoid prolonging suffering without meaningful recovery. These decisions should be made through shared decision-making and documented clearly in forms like the Physician Orders for Life-Sustaining Treatment (POLST) or advance directives. These documents provide comprehensive instructions about a patient's preferences, including whether to receive mechanical ventilation, vasopressors, or ICU care, helping to reduce interventions that conflict with their goals of care. Clinical studies have shown that patients with documented preferences often choose to forgo vasopressors and other invasive interventions, consistent with a broader limitation on life-sustaining treatment beyond CPR.[14–20]

10.4.2.2 Do Not Intubate (DNI)

Do Not Intubate refers to a decision to forgo endotracheal intubation and mechanical ventilation in the event of respiratory failure. This is particularly relevant in patients with underlying terminal illnesses, progressive frailty, or poor baseline functional status, where intubation may prolong suffering without improving quality of life. Importantly, DNI does not imply withholding all treatments; many such patients can still receive noninvasive support and symptom management.[21]

10.4.2.3 Do Not Escalate Care (DNC)

Do Not Escalate Care (DNC) encompasses broader decisions such as forgoing ICU admission, renal replacement therapy, or vasopressor support in patients with poor prognosis. This approach may be applied when aggressive interventions are unlikely to provide meaningful benefit, and when a shift toward comfort-focused care is appropriate. The DNC concept, while less formalized than DNR/DNI, is gaining traction in critical care as clinicians increasingly recognize the importance of proportional care.[22]

These decisions must be made through structured family meetings involving physicians, nurses, and palliative care teams. Effective communication should include a discussion of prognosis, likely outcomes, treatment burdens, and available alternatives. Cultural, religious, and psychosocial factors must be considered to ensure decisions reflect the patient's beliefs and values.

A parallel focus is ensuring a high quality of dying, particularly when curative options are no longer appropriate. The Quality of Dying and Death (QODD) framework includes domains such as symptom control, emotional support, communication, dignity, and spiritual care. Integrating palliative care can help manage dyspnea, anxiety, and terminal agitation in patients with end-stage pneumonia. Facilitating the presence of family members, enabling final conversations, and honoring spiritual or cultural rites are also key components.[23,24] Incorporating palliative principles into the care of severe pneumonia patients not only improves the quality of dying but also reduces moral distress among staff and improves bereavement outcomes for families.

10.5 Implementation Considerations

Effective integration includes the use of clinical triggers (e.g., ventilator support >48h, high frailty index) for referral, standardized order sets that include palliative and rehab consults, and family-centered care conferences. These practices are supported by ICU and palliative care guidelines.[11,12,25]

10.6 Conclusion

In the care of patients with severe pneumonia, the integration of palliative care and physical rehabilitation is essential. These approaches improve not only clinical outcomes but also the overall experience of care. A patient-centered model that includes both services from the early phase of illness can reduce suffering, improve recovery, and ensure that care remains aligned with the goals and values of the patient and their family.

References

1. Torres A, Niederman MS, Chastre J, et al. International guidelines for management of HAP and VAP. *Eur Respir J*. 2017;50(3):1700582.
2. Phua J, Weng L, Ling L, et al. Intensive care management of COVID-19: Challenges and recommendations. *Lancet Respir Med*. 2020;8(5):506–517.
3. WHO. Palliative care fact sheet. 2020. Available from: https://www.who.int/news-room/fact-sheets/detail/palliative-care
4. Curtis JR, Kross EK, Stapleton RD. Importance of advance care planning in critical care. *JAMA*. 2020; 323(18):1771–1772.
5. Schweickert WD, Pohlman MC, Pohlman AS, et al. Early PT in critically ill patients. *Lancet*. 2009;373(9678): 1874–82.
6. Needham DM, Davidson J, Cohen H, et al. Improving long-term ICU outcomes. *Crit Care Med*. 2012;40(2): 502–509.
7. Schweickert WD, Pohlman MC, Pohlman AS, Nigos C, Pawlik AJ, Esbrook CL, et al. Early physical and occupational therapy in mechanically ventilated, critically ill patients: A randomized controlled trial. *Lancet*. 2009;373(9678):1874–1882.
8. Hodgson CL, Berney S, Harrold M, Saxena M, Bellomo R, Cameron P, et al. Clinical review: Early patient mobilization in the ICU. *Crit Care*. 2013;17(1):207.
9. McDonald CF, Whyte K, Jenkins S, Serginson J, Frith P, Wood-Baker R, et al. Clinical practice guideline on domiciliary oxygen therapy from the Thoracic Society of Australia and New Zealand. *Respirology*. 2016;21(5):896–909.
10. Rochester CL, Vogiatzis I, Holland AE, Lareau SC, Marciniuk DD, Puhan MA, et al. An official American Thoracic Society/European Respiratory Society policy statement: Enhancing implementation, use, and delivery of pulmonary rehabilitation. *Am J Respir Crit Care Med*. 2015;192(11):1373–1386.
11. Aslakson RA, Curtis JR, Nelson JE. Changing role of palliative care in ICU. *Crit Care Med*. 2014;42(11):2418–2428.

12. Quill TE, Abernethy AP. Generalist plus specialist palliative care: Creating a more sustainable model. *N Engl J Med.* 2013;368(13):1173–1175.
13. Nelson JE, Bassett R, Boss RD, Brasel KJ, Campbell ML, Cortez TB, et al. Models for structuring a clinical initiative to enhance palliative care in the ICU: A report from the Improving Palliative Care in the ICU (IPAL-ICU) Project. *Crit Care Med.* 2010;38(9):1765–1772.
14. Lee RY, Brumback LC, Sathitratanacheewin S, et al. Association of physician orders for life-sustaining treatment with ICU admission among patients hospitalized near the end of life. *JAMA.* 2020;323(10):950–960. doi:10.1001/jama.2019.22523
15. Truog RD, Fried TR. Physician orders for life-sustaining treatment and limiting overtreatment at the end of life. *JAMA.* 2020;323(10):934–935. doi:10.1001/jama.2019.22522
16. Lee RY, Brumback LC, Sathitratanacheewin S, et al. Conflicting orders in physician orders for life-sustaining treatment forms. *J Am Geriatr Soc.* 2020;68(3):526–533. doi:10.1111/jgs.16828
17. Kim H, Kim Y, Kim K, et al. Characteristics and outcomes of patients with do-not-resuscitate and physician orders for life-sustaining treatment in a medical intensive care unit: A retrospective cohort study. *BMC Palliat Care.* 2024;23(1):42. doi:10.1186/s12904-024-01375-w
18. Jennings LA, Zingmond D, Wenger NS, et al. Care preferences in physician orders for life sustaining treatment in California nursing homes. *J Am Geriatr Soc.* 2022;70(7):2040–2050. doi:10.1111/jgs.17737
19. Silva RS, de Lima LD, Nunes NA, et al. Cross-cultural adaptation of the Physician Orders for Life-Sustaining Treatment form to Brazil. *J Palliat Med.* 2019;22(1):69–74. doi:10.1089/jpm.2017.0590
20. Hickman SE, Keevern E, Hammes BJ. Use of the Physician Orders for Life-Sustaining Treatment Program in the clinical setting: A systematic review of the literature. *J Am Geriatr Soc.* 2015;63(2):341–350. doi:10.1111/jgs.13248
21. Cook D, Rocker G. Dying with dignity in the intensive care unit. *N Engl J Med.* 2014;370(26):2506–14.
22. Hua M, Wunsch H. Integrating palliative care in the ICU. *Curr Opin Crit Care.* 2014;20(6):673–80.

23. Downey L, Engelberg RA, Curtis JR, Lafferty WE, Jarvik JG, Ludman E, et al. Shared decision-making and the quality of end-of-life care. *J Am Geriatr Soc.* 2010;58(7):1215–20.
24. Curtis JR, Downey L, Engleberg RA. The quality of dying and death: Developing a measure. *Arch Intern Med.* 2001;161(10):1211–7.
25. Spruit MA, Singh SJ, Garvey C, et al. An official ATS/ERS policy statement: Key concepts and advances in pulmonary rehabilitation. *Am J Respir Crit Care Med.* 2013; 188(8):e13–64.

Chapter 11

Vaccination

A Preventive Shield

11.1 Introduction

Pneumonia continues to be a major public health concern worldwide, contributing significantly to hospitalizations and deaths, particularly among infants and the elderly. Vaccination against common respiratory pathogens has shown substantial success in reducing disease burden.[1,2]

11.2 Vaccine-Preventable Causes of Pneumonia

The key pathogens responsible for vaccine-preventable pneumonia include *Streptococcus pneumoniae, Haemophilus influenzae* type b (Hib), influenza viruses, and SARS-CoV-2. These organisms are major contributors to both community-acquired pneumonia and severe community-acquired respiratory infections (sCAR).[3,4]

In addition, *respiratory syncytial virus* (RSV) has emerged as a significant cause of lower respiratory tract infections, especially in infants and the elderly. Although neonates are too young to receive direct RSV immunization, maternal vaccination with the RSVpreF vaccine during pregnancy confers passive immunity to newborns

 DOI:10.1201/9781003629504-11

via transplacental transfer of neutralizing antibodies.[5] For adults, Advisory Committee on Immunization Practices (ACIP) now recommends a single dose of RSV vaccine for individuals aged 60 years and older with specific risk factors such as chronic lung or heart disease, diabetes, or immunocompromised states. Additionally, adults aged 75 years and older may receive the vaccine regardless of comorbidities, and recent expansions include high-risk individuals aged 50–59 years.[6]

Herpes Zoster, resulting from reactivation of the varicella-zoster virus, is also associated with pulmonary complications, including viral pneumonia, particularly in immunocompromised individuals and patients with chronic lung diseases such as COPD. Vaccination with recombinant zoster vaccine (RZV) has been shown to reduce incidence of herpes zoster and its complications, making it relevant for this population.[7]

11.3 Immunological Mechanisms of Vaccine Protection

Pneumococcal conjugate vaccines (PCVs) induce robust T-cell-dependent immune responses by promoting antigen presentation and memory B-cell formation, providing long-term protection, especially in young children and older adults.[8] Influenza and COVID-19 vaccines stimulate both mucosal and systemic immunity, limiting viral replication and providing partial cross-protection against other respiratory viruses.[9]

The newly developed RSV vaccines, such as the bivalent pre-fusion F protein-based RSVpreF vaccine, are designed to elicit high titers of neutralizing antibodies. When administered to pregnant women, the vaccine promotes transplacental transfer of maternal antibodies to the infant, providing effective short-term protection during early infancy. The formulation includes adjuvants that enhance immunogenicity and antibody longevity.[5,10] In adults, RSV vaccines have demonstrated high efficacy in preventing lower respiratory tract disease in older adults and those with chronic medical conditions, providing another tool for pneumonia prevention in high-risk populations.[6]

The recombinant zoster vaccine (RZV; Varicella Zoster Vaccine Recombinant), which contains glycoprotein E and the AS01B adjuvant system, induces strong CD4+ T-cell responses and is highly effective in preventing zoster and zoster-related complications, even in immunocompromised and older populations. This immunological approach is crucial in reducing herpes zoster-associated pneumonia and systemic inflammation in COPD patients.[7,11]

11.4 Global Guidelines: ACIP (Advisory Committee on Immunization Practices)

ACIP, under the Centers for Disease Control and Prevention (CDC), provides annual, evidence-based vaccination schedules for children and adults in the United States. These recommendations are based on epidemiological data, vaccine efficacy, and public health priorities.[5]

11.5 ACIP Recommendations for Pneumonia Prevention: Children (0–18 years)

- PCV13 or PCV15: 4 doses at 2, 4, 6, and 12–15 months.
- Hib vaccine: 3–4 doses depending on product type.
- Influenza: Annually starting at 6 months.
- COVID-19: From 6 months of age, adjusted to current variant recommendations.
- RSV: Single dose of nirsevimab for all infants younger than 8 months born during or entering their first RSV season. For high-risk infants aged 8–19 months, a second season dose may be considered.[12]

11.6 Adults (≥19 years)

- PCV20, or PCV15 followed by PPSV23, especially for those ≥65 years or with chronic conditions.
- Influenza: Yearly for all adults.
- COVID-19: Primary and booster doses depending on variant and exposure risk.
- RSV: A single dose for adults aged ≥60 years based on shared clinical decision-making, especially for those with chronic conditions or residing in long-term care facilities. Adults aged ≥75 years or high-risk individuals aged 50–59 years may also be considered.[6]

ACIP guidelines are widely regarded for their systematic review methodology and their role in guiding national immunization programs.[9]

11.7 National Guidelines for Vaccination

In addition to ACIP in the United States, several countries and regions have developed their own immunization guidelines tailored to their epidemiological context, healthcare infrastructure, and population needs. For example, the European Centre for Disease Prevention and Control (ECDC) coordinates immunization programs across EU member states, and in Asia, countries like Japan, South Korea, and Indonesia have established comprehensive national vaccination guidelines.

In Indonesia, the Indonesian Society of Internal Medicine (*Perhimpunan Dokter Spesialis Penyakit Dalam Indonesia*, PAPDI) issues recommendations for adult immunization, including pneumococcal, influenza, herpes zoster, COVID-19, and RSV vaccines, especially for elderly individuals and those with comorbid conditions. PAPDI plays a crucial role in aligning national vaccination practices with global standards and adapting them to local disease burdens.

These national guidelines provide context-specific recommendations that complement global strategies, ensuring effective and equitable protection against vaccine-preventable respiratory diseases (Table 11.1).

11.8 Impact of Vaccination on Pneumonia and sCAR Burden

Introduction of PCV has reduced invasive pneumococcal disease (IPD) and hospitalizations for pneumonia by up to 50%. Hib and influenza vaccines have substantially lowered rates of secondary bacterial pneumonia. COVID-19 vaccines have significantly reduced rates of viral pneumonia and ARDS in both adult and pediatric populations.[6]

The recent inclusion of RSV vaccination has demonstrated reduction in RSV-related hospitalizations among infants through maternal immunization, and in older adults and high-risk populations such as those with COPD. RSV vaccines also help reduce severe exacerbations and secondary infections in these groups. Similarly, the recombinant zoster vaccine (RZV) has shown benefit in reducing herpes zoster complications, including zoster-associated pneumonia in immunocompromised and COPD patients, further supporting its role in decreasing sCAR burden in vulnerable populations.[13,14]

11.9 Challenges and Future Perspectives

Despite proven vaccine effectiveness, challenges remain, including vaccine hesitancy due to misinformation and cultural beliefs, which reduce vaccine uptake. Inequitable vaccine access, especially in resource-limited settings, further widens disparities. Moreover, adult immunization is often underused because healthcare providers may

TABLE 11.1 Comparative Recommendations for Pneumonia-Related Vaccinations in Selected Regions

Region	Pneumococcal	Influenza	COVID-19	RSV	Herpes Zoster
United States	PCV13/15/20 + PPSV23	Annual	Primary + boosters	Adults ≥60 y (shared decision), infants (maternal/nirsevimab)	Adults ≥50 y (RZV)
Europe (ECDC)	PCV13 or 23-valent	Annual	National plans vary	Adults ≥60 y, some countries recommend maternal vaccine	Adults ≥60 y (varies)
Indonesia (PAPDI)	PCV13/PCV15+ PPSV23 PCV20	Annual	National schedule	High Risk Adults ≥50 y, recommend maternal vaccine (non adjuvant)	Adults ≥50 y (RZV)

Abbreviations: ACIP: Advisory Committee on Immunization Practices; CDC: Centers for Disease Control and Prevention; ECDC: European Centre for Disease Prevention and Control; PAPDI: Perhimpunan Dokter Spesialis Penyakit Dalam Indonesia; PCV: Pneumococcal Conjugate Vaccine; PPSV: Pneumococcal Polysaccharide Vaccine; RSV: Respiratory Syncytial Virus; RZV: Recombinant Zoster Vaccine.

lack sufficient time or training to educate and encourage patients about vaccines, leading to lower acceptance.

Future prospects include the introduction of higher-valency pneumococcal vaccines such as PCV21, development of mucosal COVID-19 vaccines to boost local immunity, and enhancements in cold-chain logistics to improve vaccine availability in low-resource areas. Educating healthcare providers to improve communication with patients on vaccination benefits is essential to increase coverage globally.[13–15]

11.10 Conclusion

Vaccination is a central pillar in pneumonia prevention strategies. Adherence to international and national guidelines can significantly reduce the burden of pneumonia and sCAR across all age groups. Strengthening public trust, improving access, and integrating vaccination in chronic disease care remains one of the goals for a better vaccination program achievement.

References

1. Andre FE, Booy R, Bock HL, Clemens J, Datta SK, John TJ, et al. Vaccination greatly reduces disease, disability, death and inequity worldwide. *Bull World Health Organ.* 2008;86(2):140–146.
2. Rudan I, Boschi-Pinto C, Biloglav Z, Mulholland K, Campbell H. Epidemiology and etiology of childhood pneumonia. *Lancet Infect Dis.* 2008;8(4):365–373.
3. Jain S, Self WH, Wunderink RG, Fakhran S, Balk R, Bramley AM, et al. Community-acquired pneumonia requiring hospitalization among U.S. adults. *N Engl J Med.* 2015;373(5):415–427.
4. Plotkin SA. Correlates of protection induced by vaccination. *Clin Vaccine Immunol.* 2008;15(3):105–109.
5. Centers for Disease Control and Prevention (CDC). Immunization schedules: United States, 2024. Available from: https://www.cdc.gov/vaccines/schedules

6. Pilishvili T, Lexau C, Farley MM, Hadler J, Harrison LH, Bennett NM, et al. Sustained reductions in invasive pneumococcal disease in the era of conjugate vaccine. *N Engl J Med.* 2010;362(5):355–365.

7. Kobayashi M, Farrar JL, Gierke R, Britton A, Leidner AJ, Romero JR, et al. Use of 15-valent and 20-valent pneumococcal conjugate vaccines among U.S. adults: Updated ACIP recommendations. *MMWR Morb Mortal Wkly Rep.* 2022;71(4):109–117.

8. CDC. Pneumococcal vaccination: Summary of who and when to vaccinate. Updated 2023. Available from: https://www.cdc.gov/vaccines/vpd/pneumo/hcp/who-when-to-vaccinate.html

9. Centers for Disease Control and Prevention. General Best Practice Guidelines for Immunization. 2023. Available from: https://www.cdc.gov/vaccines/hcp/acip-recs/general-recs/index.html

10. Perhimpunan Dokter Spesialis Penyakit Dalam Indonesia (PAPDI). *Rekomendasi imunisasi dewasa.* Jakarta: PAPDI; 2022.

11. Kementerian Kesehatan Republik Indonesia. *Strategi Nasional Vaksinasi COVID-19 dan Influenza.* Jakarta: Kemenkes RI; 2023.

12. PAPDI. *Update imunisasi dewasa nasional.* Jakarta: PAPDI; 2023.

13. Pilishvili T, Lexau C, Farley MM, Hadler J, Harrison LH, Bennett NM, et al. Sustained reductions in invasive pneumococcal disease in the era of conjugate vaccine. *N Engl J Med.* 2010;362(5):355–365.

14. Nohynek H, Wilder-Smith A. Does the World Still Need New Vaccines Against Pneumonia? *Lancet Infect Dis.* 2017;17(11):1120–1121.

15. World Health Organization. *Immunization Agenda 2030: A Global Strategy to Leave No One Behind.* Geneva: WHO; 2020.

CHAPTER 12

A Case-Based Perspective on Severe Pneumonia in Immunocompromised Patients

12.1 Introduction

Immunocompromised patients—those with primary immunodeficiencies, solid or hematologic malignancies, autoimmune conditions requiring immunosuppressants, or those undergoing chemotherapy or transplantation—constitute a uniquely vulnerable group with altered pulmonary defense mechanisms.[1,2]

Pneumonia in these patients is frequently polymicrobial, rapidly progressive, and associated with high morbidity and mortality. The diagnostic yield of conventional microbiologic methods is often suboptimal due to prior antimicrobial exposure, low organism burden, or nonbacterial pathogens.[3] Early and precise diagnosis is critical, as delayed or empirical treatment may fail to cover atypical organisms or MDR strains.

Moreover, altered inflammatory responses in these patients may blunt typical clinical features or radiographic

DOI:10.1201/9781003629504-12

findings, further complicating diagnosis.[4] A multidisciplinary approach, including early bronchoscopy, use of multiplex molecular panels, and strict vaccination protocols, is essential to optimize outcomes.[5]

CASE 1   EARLY BRONCHOSCOPY AND PATHOGEN DETECTION IN A CVID PATIENT

A 47-year-old male with Common Variable Immunodeficiency (CVID), neurogenic dysphagia, and chronic tracheostomy was admitted for progressive dyspnea. On day 3 of hospitalization, he developed acute respiratory failure requiring mechanical ventilation. A high-resolution chest computed tomography (CT) scan revealed bilateral consolidations and centrilobular nodules. Bronchoscopy with bronchoalveolar lavage (BAL), performed within 24 hours of intubation, identified *ESBL-producing Escherichia coli*, *Klebsiella pneumoniae*, and *Candida tropicalis*.

Targeted antibiotic and antifungal treatment resulted in rapid clinical improvement and discharge by day 14.

Discussion

This case illustrates the importance of early bronchoscopy in immunocompromised hosts, particularly those with suspected polymicrobial infections. Patients with CVID lack effective IgG-mediated opsonization, rendering them susceptible to encapsulated and Gram-negative organisms.[6] Tracheostomy and dysphagia increase the risk of aspiration and colonization by hospital-acquired flora.[7]

BAL within 24–48 hours of intubation has been associated with significantly higher diagnostic yields and lower mortality, particularly when guided by rapid molecular panels.[8,9] FilmArray Pneumonia Panel and other syndromic assays can detect bacteria, viruses, fungi, and resistance genes within hours, allowing precise de-escalation or escalation of therapy (Figures 12.1 and 12.2).[10]

Detection Summary						
Bacteria						
				Bin (copies/mL)		
	Bin (copies/mL)		10^4	10^5	10^6	≥10^7
Detected: ✓	10^5	*Enterobacter cloacae* complex				
✓	10^5	*Klebsiella pneumoniae* group				
✓	10^4	*Acinetobacter calcoaceticus-baumannii* complex				

⚠ Note: Detection of bacterial nucleic acid may be indicative of colonizing or normal respiratory flora and may not indicate the causative agent of pneumonia. Semi-quantitative Bin (copies/mL) results generated by the FilmArray Pneumonia Panel *plus* are not equivalent to CFU/mL and do not consistently correlate with the quantity of bacterial analytes compared to CFU/mL. For specimens with multiple bacteria detected, the relative abundance of nucleic acids (copies/mL) may not correlate with the relative abundance of bacteria as determined by culture (CFU/mL). Clinical correlation is advised to determine significance of semi-quantitative Bin (copies/mL) for clinical management.

Antimicrobial Resistance Genes
Detected: ✓ CTX-M

⚠ Note: Antimicrobial resistance can occur via multiple mechanisms. A Not Detected result for a genetic marker of antimicrobial resistance does not indicate susceptibility to associated antimicrobial drugs or drug classes. A Detected result for a genetic marker of antimicrobial resistance cannot be definitively linked to the microorganism(s) detected. Culture is required to obtain isolates for antimicrobial susceptibility testing and FilmArray Pneumonia Panel *plus* results should be used in conjunction with culture results for the determination of susceptibility or resistance.

Atypical Bacteria
Detected: None

Viruses
Detected: ✓ Respiratory Syncytial Virus

FIGURE 12.1 FilmArray Pneumonia Panel output from BAL specimen in CVID case. Shows multiplex detection of *Klebsiella pneumoniae* with CTX-M gene, *E. coli*, and *Candida tropicalis*—prompting early targeted therapy.

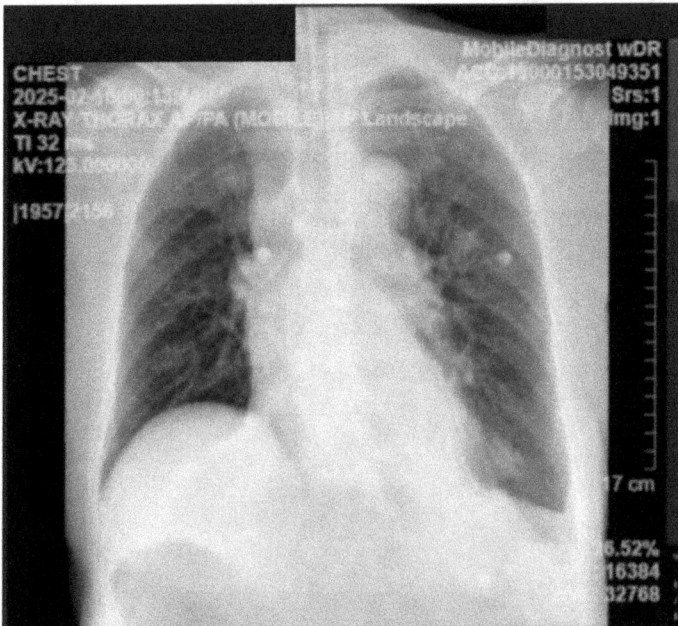

FIGURE 12.2 Chest radiograph (AP view) from Case 1 on Day 2 of mechanical ventilation. Demonstrates bilateral opacities and air bronchograms. The radiographic picture supported clinical suspicion for polymicrobial infection.

CASE 2   FATAL POLYMICROBIAL PNEUMONIA IN A PATIENT WITH METASTATIC LUNG CANCER

A 75-year-old female with stage IV lung adenocarcinoma on targeted EGFR-TKI therapy presented with a vesicular rash, cough, and low-grade fever. She had not received recent pneumococcal, influenza, or varicella-zoster vaccines. Chest imaging showed diffuse infiltrates and pleural effusion. She deteriorated rapidly despite broad-spectrum empiric therapy and died within 72 hours due to refractory septic shock and multi-organ failure.

Discussion

This case reflects the deadly synergy of viral–bacterial coinfection and unvaccinated status in an immunocompromised host. Reactivated varicella-zoster virus (VZV) and secondary bacterial pneumonia can rapidly progress in oncology patients with reduced T-cell immunity. EGFR-TKIs are known to impair immune surveillance and epithelial repair, further compounding risk.[11]

Missed vaccinations in cancer patients remain common due to fragmented care, fear of vaccine-induced side effects, and lack of standardized oncology-immunization protocols.[12,13] Proactive vaccination against influenza, pneumococcus, and now RSV is essential, as endorsed by both the Centers for Disease Control and Prevention (CDC) and National Comprehensive Cancer Network (NCCN) guidelines.[14,15]

12.2 Viral–Bacterial Coinfections: RSV as a Paradigm

Respiratory syncytial virus (RSV) has emerged as a key viral pathogen causing severe pneumonia in older and immunocompromised adults. Beyond direct viral injury, RSV infection disrupts epithelial integrity and innate immunity, facilitating secondary bacterial invasion—particularly by *Streptococcus pneumoniae, Haemophilus influenzae,* and *Staphylococcus aureus.*[16,17]

A 2025 JAMA study demonstrated RSV vaccine effectiveness (VE) of 67–73% in immunocompromised adults, reducing hospitalization and mortality significantly.[18] FDA approval of newer RSV vaccines (e.g., mRESVIA by Moderna) has expanded access to adults aged 18–59 with comorbidities.[19]

12.3 The Role of Host Cellular Immunity

Immunocompromised patients not only face microbial threats but also dysregulated immune responses. A prospective BAL study found that low CD4+ T-cell counts in lavage fluid were independently associated with extubation failure and in-ICU mortality.[20] Alterations in alveolar macrophage function, neutrophil extracellular trap (NET) dysregulation, and suppressed interferon signaling have also been implicated.[21,22] These findings suggest that pneumonia outcomes are not solely pathogen-driven but also shaped by host immune capacity.

12.4 Prevention and Syndromic Diagnosis: The Integrated Approach

These two cases illustrate dual imperatives in managing severe pneumonia in immunocompromised patients:

1. Early, pathogen-directed diagnosis using bronchoscopy + molecular panels: Enables precision therapy, avoids overuse of broad-spectrum agents, and improves outcomes.
2. Vaccination against preventable pathogens (pneumococcus, influenza, RSV, VZV): Reduces incidence, severity, and mortality of pneumonia in high-risk populations.

ATS/IDSA guidelines now support early bronchoscopy in undiagnosed severe CAP, especially in patients at risk for MDR or opportunistic infections.[23] Meanwhile, immunization guidelines by CDC/ACIP and NCCN emphasize adult vaccination even during cancer therapy or chronic immunosuppression.[14,15,24]

12.5 Conclusion

Severe pneumonia in immunocompromised individuals requires a paradigm shift—from empirical, reactive treatment to early, personalized, and preventive strategies. Timely bronchoscopy, molecular diagnostics, and adherence to adult vaccination schedules represent critical pillars of care. As pathogens evolve and immunity profiles shift, integrating diagnostics with immunoprophylaxis will be the key to improving outcomes in this vulnerable population (Table 12.1).

TABLE 12.1 Common Pathogens, Diagnostic Modalities, and Preventive Measures in Immunocompromised Patients with Severe Pneumonia

Pathogen Type	Examples	Risk Group	Preferred Diagnostic	Prevention (if available)
Bacterial (MDR)	*Pseudomonas aeruginosa*, ESBL-*E. coli*, *Klebsiella pneumoniae*, MRSA	CVID, cancer, ICU patients with prior antibiotics	BAL + culture ± multiplex PCR (e.g. FilmArray)	Pneumococcal vaccine (PCV20, PPSV23)
Opportunistic Fungi	*Candida* spp., *Aspergillus* spp., *Pneumocystis jirovecii*	CVID, transplant, prolonged neutropenia	BAL + fungal stain, Galactomannan, PCR	No vaccine; chemoprophylaxis in select cases
Viruses (Respiratory)	RSV, Influenza A/B, SARS-CoV-2, CMV, VZV	Older adults, cancer therapy, transplant	NP/OP swab or BAL multiplex PCR	Influenza, RSV, COVID-19, VZV vaccines
Polymicrobial	RSV + *S. pneumoniae*, Influenza + MRSA	Elderly, EGFR-TKI, CVID, HIV	Syndromic panel on BAL or ETA	Combined vaccine strategies + early diagnosis

References

1. Bonilla FA, Barlan I, Chapel H, et al. ICON: Common variable immunodeficiency disorders. *J Allergy Clin Immunol Pract.* 2016;4(1):38–59.
2. CDC. Pneumococcal vaccination: Summary of who and when to vaccinate. Updated October 2023.
3. Martinez RM, et al. Diagnostic yield of bronchoscopy with BAL in immunocompromised patients. *Chest.* 2020;158(6):2458–2467.
4. De Pauw BE. Infectious complications in patients with neutropenia. *Curr Opin Infect Dis.* 2022;35(6):531–537.
5. Torres A, et al. The role of bronchoscopy in managing severe pneumonia in ICU patients. *Intensive Care Med.* 2019;45(5):567–579.
6. Cunningham-Rundles C. Common variable immune deficiency: Dissection of the variable. *Immunol Rev.* 2019;287(1):145–161.
7. Raghu G, et al. Respiratory tract colonization and risk of infection in patients with tracheostomy. *Clin Respir J.* 2020;14(5):400–408.
8. Huang L, et al. Fiberoptic bronchoscopy and BAL in immunocompromised ICU patients: Safety and diagnostic value. *Respir Care.* 2021;66(3):453–460.
9. Kim Y, et al. BAL microbiological yield and management change in immunocompromised pneumonia. *BMC Pulm Med.* 2022;22:143.
10. Babady NE, et al. Multiplex PCR in respiratory tract infections: Impact on antimicrobial stewardship. *Clin Microbiol Rev.* 2022;35(1):e00203–e00221.
11. Masood A, et al. EGFR tyrosine kinase inhibitors and infection risk in lung cancer patients. *J Thorac Oncol.* 2023;18(2):189–197.
12. O'Halloran AC, et al. Missed opportunities for adult vaccination in cancer patients. *Am J Prev Med.* 2020;58(6):e155–e163.
13. Baden LR, et al. Prevention and treatment of cancer-related infections: NCCN Guidelines v2.2022. *J Natl Compr Canc Netw.* 2022;20(4):384–406.
14. CDC. RSV Vaccination for Adults. Updated October 2023.

15. FDA. Press Release: Approval of mRESVIA for at-risk adults aged 18–59. June 2025.
16. Falsey AR, et al. Respiratory syncytial virus—associated illness in adults with advanced COPD and/or CHF. *J Infect Dis.* 2021;223(3):416–426.
17. Talbot HK, et al. RSV hospitalization and vaccine effectiveness in adults ≥60: a real-world study. *JAMA Netw Open.* 2025;8(5):e2512345.
18. Fry SE, Terebuh P, Kaelber DC, Xu R, Davis PB. Effectiveness and safety of respiratory syncytial virus vaccine for US adults aged 60 years or older. JAMA Netw Open. 2025;8(5):e258322. doi:10.1001/jamanetworkopen.2025.8322
19. He Y, et al. BAL lymphocyte subsets and extubation failure in severe pneumonia. *BMC Pulm Med.* 2023;23:212.
20. Ritchie AI, et al. Host–pathogen interactions in immunocompromised lung infections. *Lancet Respir Med.* 2023;11(4):350–362.
21. Dickson RP, et al. Lung microbiota and host response in immunosuppression. *Am J Respir Crit Care Med.* 2022;205(6):651–660.
22. Metlay JP, et al. ATS/IDSA CAP guidelines. *Am J Respir Crit Care Med.* 2019;200(7):e45–e67.
23. NCCN. Adult Immunization in Oncology. Version 1. 2024.
24. ACIP. *Adult Immunization Schedule*: United States, 2024.

Index

Pages in *italics* refer to figures and pages in **bold** refer to tables.

For Product Safety Concerns and Information please contact our EU
representative GPSR@taylorandfrancis.com
Taylor & Francis Verlag GmbH, Kaufingerstraße 24, 80331 München, Germany